Resilience and Well-being for Dental Professionals

Mahrukh Khwaja
Dentist and Positive Psychologist
UK

WILEY Blackwell

Registered Offices
John Wiley & Sons, Inc., 111 River Street, Hoboken, NJ 07030, USA
John Wiley & Sons Ltd, The Atrium, Southern Gate, Chichester, West Sussex, PO19 8SQ, UK

For details of our global editorial offices, customer services, and more information about Wiley products visit us at www.wiley.com.

Wiley also publishes its books in a variety of electronic formats and by print-on-demand. Some content that appears in standard print versions of this book may not be available in other formats.

Library of Congress Cataloging-in-Publication Data
Names: Khwaja, Mahrukh, author.
Title: Resilience and well-being for dental professionals / Mahrukh Khwaja.
Description: Hoboken, NJ : Wiley, 2023. | Includes bibliographical
    references and index.
Identifiers: LCCN 2022031398 (print) | LCCN 2022031399 (ebook) | ISBN
    9781119814504 (paperback) | ISBN 9781119814511 (adobe pdf) | ISBN
    9781119814528 (epub)
Subjects: MESH: Dentists–psychology | Resilience, Psychological | Burnout,
    Professional–prevention & control
Classification: LCC RK53 (print) | LCC RK53 (ebook) | NLM WU 21 | DDC
    617.6001/9–dc23/eng/20220801
LC record available at https://lccn.loc.gov/2022031398
LC ebook record available at https://lccn.loc.gov/2022031399

Cover Design: Wiley
Cover Image: Courtesy of Mahrukh Khwaja

Set in 9.5/12.5pt STIXTwoText by Straive, Pondicherry, India

Contents

Foreword

The health and well-being of members of the dental team is of paramount importance, and yet there is abundant evidence that working within dentistry has a profound negative impact. There is an unforgivable paucity of research exploring the experience of members of the dental team other than dentists; however, a comprehensive review by Plessas et al (2021) identifies not only a comprehensive range of factors that impinge upon the well-being of dentists but suggests from a review of previous studies that between 60% and 80% of dentists experience significant levels of burnout. The moral imperative to support and assist individuals is clear. Additionally, there is strong evidence that clinicians experiencing such high levels of burnout are more likely to leave the profession, adding to the challenge of access to dental services faced in many countries, and are at increased risk of making errors that have harmful effects for their patients (Hodkinson et al 2022).

To date there has been no comprehensive publication that has sought to provide guidance on addressing the stress of dental practice and its impact on mental health and well-being. Mahrukh Khwaja has provided such a guidebook informed uniquely by her experience as a dental practitioner. I recommend it to all involved in the practice of dentistry.

It may at first appear that there is much to do and much to learn in this comprehensive book. The key is to make small changes that accumulate. Find one thing that you think you are able to undertake, and work with that. As you begin to take control of your well-being, you will find that change becomes easier. Keep this book with you as a manual for working in dentistry. Looking after yourself is equally important as your development and maintenance of the clinical skills of dentistry. I hope this book supports you in your journey to finding (or re-finding) the joy of practicing dentistry, caring for others, and helping them to achieve the benefits of oral health. Good luck.

Tim Newton
King's College London

References

Hodkinson, A., Zhou, A., Johnson, J., Geraghty, K., Riley, R., et al. (2022). Associations of physician burnout with career engagement and quality of patient care: systematic review and meta-analysis. *BMJ*; 378: e070442.

Plessas, A., Paisi, M., Bryce, M., Burns, L., O'Brien, T., Witton, R., and Hanoch, Y. (2021). Mental health and wellbeing in dentistry: a rapid evidence assessment. General Dental Council.

Preface

In my 12 years of clinical practice as a general Dental Practitioner, I have experienced burnout multiple times. Despite dually qualifying in Dentistry with a Psychology BSc, and having a good theoretical understanding of mental illness, it was not until I experienced my personal journey of reduced resilience levels and poor mental well-being that I fully appreciated the toll and stigma attached with it. This insight and my curiosity ultimately lead me to find a powerful calling: a mission to bring preventative solutions to the heart of the mental health conversation in dentistry.

As I explored mental health support in dentistry, whilst completing my Master's in Applied Positive Psychology, I realised that although there were services for crisis point, there were no clinician-orientated preventative programmes to help us before we are ill. Clinician well-being training still remains largely missing from the undergraduate curriculum and the postgraduate agenda, with much of the focus solely on clinical competency. This imbalance in clinical education in dentistry needs urgent addressing. Without a doubt, we are currently facing a global mental health crisis, one where understanding the tools means we are much more able to cope and, further still, thrive during challenges in dentistry.

The aetiology of poor mental health in dentistry is complex and multifactorial. The solutions need to take a broad approach also: moving away from solely crisis point to considering the role of prevention.

This book is designed with prevention in mind. My intention is to break down the key psychological well-being theories, connect them with dentistry, and help you apply them to your life. A big part of your own resilience and well-being journey is to firstly develop self-awareness and then experiment with the evidence-based tools. See which practices fit you the best and remain actively engaged with building positive health.

The big idea I came across in my research for preventative solutions is that just like we exercise our physical body and its muscles, the brain needs to exercise. Each chapter has brain workout exercises to help you build the muscles of happiness, gratitude, self-compassion, growth mindset, grit, and resilience and help you practice them consistently. Beyond reducing anxiety and depressive feelings, this book is a self-intervention: a self-help companion in enhancing your positive emotions, life satisfaction, growing optimism, purpose, mindset, nurturing positive relationships, and living a rich and meaningful life as a dental professional. To flourish in dentistry.

The tone of this book very much aligns with my values: kindness, compassion, warmth, and empathy. I have lived the mental health crises explored in this book, and this insight informs my passion for creating the book. As with learning any tools, give yourself plenty of self-love and room for setbacks. Building resilience and well-being whilst balancing a busy dental career and a personal life is not a linear journey. Approaching the tools with compassion first is key.

Leaning into the knowledge that despite adversities and life's invariable bumps, we can train ourselves to become more resilient and be the creators of an optimistic future in dentistry is the challenge. Welcome to an exhilarating self-development journey!

Dr Mahrukh Khwaja BDS PGCert (Aesthetic Dentistry)
BSc Psychology MAPP

About the Author

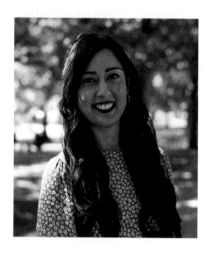

Dr Mahrukh Khwaja is a Dentist, Positive Psychologist, accredited mindfulness teacher, and the founder of Mind Ninja, a first-of-its-kind wellness start-up dedicated to improving mental health and resilience among dental professionals.

With more than 12 years of clinical experience 'at the chair-side', Dr Khwaja has an insider's perspective on the unique stressors affecting dental professionals. She also has firsthand knowledge of the lack of industry-specific mental health tools and support – something she discovered during her own bout with burnout. With nothing of its kind currently available in the dental industry, she envisioned a system of support that, just like daily flossing and brushing, took a preventive maintenance approach to mental health. Drawing on the neuroscience of well-being and positive psychology, she developed Mind Ninja as a solution that would help fellow dental professionals build mental resilience, foster connection and meaning, and thrive.

Mind Ninja offers a comprehensive range of training, coaching, and wellness products that go beyond reducing symptoms of stress to generating a solid foundation of positive well-being. These tools are designed to help dental professionals thrive in any environment, ensuring that their own bright smiles come from a place of genuine mental health. Dr Khwaja has delivered Mind Ninja's bespoke workshops and well-being programmes to bring transformative change to a diverse range of organisations, including Unilever, Colgate, NHS Oxford Health, King's College London, Acteon, British Dental Association, and the Royal College of Physicians and Surgeons of Glasgow. Mind Ninja received Global Health Pharma's 2022 Award for Excellence in Innovation and was a shortlisted finalist at the Private Dentistry Awards in 2021 and 2020.

Mind Ninja's flagship wellness product is the *Mind Flossing Toolkit*. This multipurpose deck of well-being cards features positive psychology interventions that inform and inspire dental professionals to build on their strengths and develop a growth mindset as well as practise mindfulness, self-compassion, and gratitude, both in the dental clinic and at home. The verdict is already in about its ability to create life-changing results: 100% of users report an improvement in their mental well-being after using the toolkit.

Dr Khwaja has been named in the *Top 50 in Dentistry* two years in a row (2022 and 2021) by FMC for her work on mental health in dentistry. Email her on mahrukh@mind-ninja.co.uk or connect with her on Instagram @mindninja.wellbeing.

Navigating Each Chapter

Each chapter has colour-coded sections that help you engage and apply the science of well-being. Try the 'Measure Your Well-being' section to measure your levels of wellness, read the 'Learning from Movies' section to see examples in popular culture, and do the 'Mind-Flossing Exercises' to build your muscles of resilience.

Chapter Overview	A quick reference summary of the topics covered in the chapter
Learning from Movies	Using pop culture references to bring alive psychology concepts and their application to the real world
Think About It	A section asking questions to help you relate the content to your own life
Measure Your Well-being	A psychological scale to measure your well-being levels

Mind-Flossing
Exercise

Activities that help you to apply what has been learnt

Mind-Flossing
Journaling Exercise

Journaling activities to help you explore the themes of the
chapter

The View from Here

Conclusion for each chapter

About the Companion Website

This book is accompanied by a companion website.

www.wiley.com/go/khwaja-resilience-dentistry

The companion website linked to this book houses all of the downloadable worksheets for you to print if needed. Guided meditations will also be found here, covering a range of topics, from a guided body scan to burnout detection and discovering your compassionate voice, to growing gratitude and honing in on strengths.

Acknowledgments

This book would not be possible without the generous contributions of many wonderful individuals. Thank you to Professor Tim Newton for sparking my interest in psychology 18 years ago as a first-year dental student at King's College London, and then championing me in taking the next steps in founding my own well-being company and creating a resilience course. Tim's advice and encouragement really helped me find the courage to step into the arena of psychology and teach in the first place.

Many of my ideas have formed from applying positive psychology in a practical sense: teaching and coaching dental professionals via workshops, well-being programmes, and products. A massive thanks to the dental organisations who gave me the opportunities to spotlight clinician well-being. I'm extremely grateful to Stancey Coughlan (commercial director, Acteon). Stancey has been a steadfast supporter and enthusiastic in advocating the health of dental professionals. I am fortunate to have met her and grateful for her continued support in all my ventures. Many thanks to the wonderful Dr Raj Jabbal and Callum Villmeter (Cephtactics) for the opportunity to bring well-being training to postgraduates and their advice on getting this book out there. Thanks to Payman Fatemi, Prav Solanki, and Shaz Memon for their support in encouraging me to keep persisting.

I am also thankful for my many mentors and coaches: from my wonderful teachers from Anglia Ruskin, particularly Bridget Grenville-Cleave; to my coach, Mariam Akhtar, for encouraging me whilst writing to lean into my strengths and inject fun; and Dr Janine Brooks MBE for her positivity around clinician well-being and kind introduction to Wiley-Blackwell.

I am grateful for my friends who reviewed drafts, provided valuable suggestions, and always championed my work. Special thanks to Robiha Nazir, Hoda Sepehrara, Raabiha Maan, Zainab Al-Mukhtar, Marjia Monsur, Maria Reza, Serwa Bayezidi, and Miglena Trangos. Deep gratitude to my friend Shabbir Mellick for giving me the confidence to dream big and write this book. It is through Shabbir's example, having written so many useful and practical books, that I had the courage to explore writing in the first instance.

A very special thanks to my amazing family: not only did they review countless iterations of this book, they also gave me the necessary emotional support to undertake this two-year project. Deep gratitude to my parents, Babra and Zahid Khwaja, who are great sources of inspiration on how to live the "good life", with my lessons on happiness, gratitude, and compassion being learnt as a young child through watching them. Grateful for my brother Zohaib for helping me work through what an ideal resilience framework for dental professionals could look like. Thank you to my brother Jahanzaib for reminding me of the power of simplifying – despite my resistance, your wisdom did sink in! Gratitude to my sister-in-law, Hena, for reminding me to inject fun into the writing process as well as helping me reframe challenges. Thanks to my then-two-year-old nephew, Zayd, for bringing much laughter and utter havoc at times, and yet reminding me of the joy of playfulness. Deep gratitude to my wonderful husband, Aniq, for helping me in so many countless ways, from cheerleading me along the way, nudging me towards an optimistic and growth mindset during testing moments, to sitting with me to bounce ideas, especially one key moment: coming up with the PERLE acronym on a midnight brainstorming session! I felt so supported and couldn't have asked for a better partnership.

Finally, thanks to the many professionals at Wiley-Blackwell involved in illustrations, editing, and publishing this book, with special thanks to my editor Monica Rogers and copyeditor Sarah Brown. Bringing these ideas to dentistry has been one of the most pivotal moments in my career. I give thanks to Wiley-Blackwell for supporting me in making this dream a reality.

1

Mental Health in Dentistry

CHAPTER OVERVIEW

- Mental health continuum
- Stressors in dentistry
- Evolutionary origins of stress
- Coping styles to stress
- Burnout and compassion fatigue
- Preventative interventions
- Measuring your stress and burnout levels.

What mental health needs is more sunlight, more candour, and more una-shamed conversation.

–Glenn Close, actress and founder of mental health charity Bring Change to Mind

A dental professional wears many hats: a mechanic, artist, educator, leader, life-long learner, sometimes a counsellor, and, at the heart of all roles, a caregiver. We are in the privileged position to help guide positive behaviour change. From building preventative oral hygiene habits to smoking cessation and reducing the frequency of sugary attacks, dental professionals are in the business of helping patients with their physical and mental well-being. The high demands on this role require considerable clinician resilience and well-being.

As dental students, one of the first pivotal principles taught to us is that prevention is better than cure. In this book, we explore exactly that: the case for clinician well-being training before we are ill. Chapter 1 kicks off this conversation with delving deep into mental health in dentistry. We explore the mental health continuum, the current mental health of dental professionals, occupational hazards, the psychology of stress, and the need to train the mind muscles.

Resilience and Well-being for Dental Professionals, First Edition. Mahrukh Khwaja.
© 2023 John Wiley & Sons Ltd. Published 2023 by John Wiley & Sons Ltd.
Companion website: www.wiley.com/go/khwaja-resilience-dentistry

Understanding the Mental Health Continuum

Mental health is a dynamic process and is always shifting. More than simply a lack of mental disorder, the World Health Organization (WHO) defines mental health as a 'state of well-being whereby individuals recognise their abilities, are able to cope with the normal stresses of life, work productively and fruitfully, and make a contribution to their communities' (WHO 2004). A crucial factor in the case for preventative clinician training is that are we are all on the mental health continuum. Imagine one end of this continuum representing minimum mental fitness (lower levels of mental health and resilience) and the other end representing maximum mental fitness (high levels of mental health and resilience). Our starting point is somewhere on this continuum dependent on our genetic makeup (see Figure 1.1).

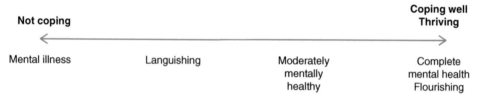

Figure 1.1 Mental health continuum.

Table 1.1 Risk and protective factors influencing our mental health.

Risk factors	Protective factors
Genetics	Self-awareness
Pessimistic thinking style	Emotional regulation
Lack of positive coping skills	Self-belief
Alcohol	Thinking flexibility
Drugs	Good nutrition
Smoking	Good sleep
Poor nutrition	Psychical exercise
Poor sleep	Mindfulness
Lack of exercise	Spirituality
Traumatic life events	Positive relationships
Negative relationships	Strong social network
Lack of social support	Meaning
Lack of meaning	Values and beliefs

Positive and negative life outcomes also impact whether we shift up and down this continuum. Both our genetics and life's events are not within our direct control. What we can influence, however, are our protective and risk factors and hence encourage a positive movement towards better mental well-being despite adversities. Table 1.1 illustrates the factors that influence mental health. While we will always be shifting up and down the continuum, we can take active steps to keep us mentally fit. This book focuses on how you can boost your levels of protective factors and encourage shifting towards maximum mental well-being.

Understanding the Stressors in Dentistry

Dentistry is a profession that is historically well known for its stressors. The origins of stress are already present, prior to qualifying. This is in part due to the high academic pressures of an intensive five-year programme paired with the early introduction of clinical care (Newton et al. 1994). Table 1.2 sums up the common factors stated in the literature.

Table 1.2   Stressors in dentistry.

- Fear of litigation
- Time pressures
- Challenging management of patients
- Administrative duties, for example, notes and referrals
- Staffing issues
- Isolation
- High workload
- Contract frustrations
- Perfectionism
- Imposter syndrome
- Social media
- Work–life balance

Collin et al. 2019; Kay and Lowe 2008; Newton et al. 2006.

Think About It

Stress is a thinking, emotional, and physical response to internal and/or external demands and pressures. It is our body's reaction to feeling under pressure. In short bursts, stress can help us meet the demands of working with patients and at home. However, chronic activation of stress impairs our health. Too much stress can affect our mood, our body, and our relationships – especially when it feels out of our control. *According to you, what are your current stress levels?*

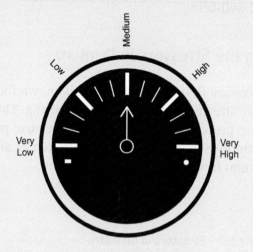

The Yerkes–Dodson Stress Performance Curve illustrates effectively how a certain amount of stress is required for our optimal performance and indeed allows us to focus and feel energised (Yerkes and Dodson 1908). Beyond the optimal level, however, and where the point of the curve starts to dip, leads us to the danger zone of fatigue, emotional exhaustion, poor health, and a phenomenon known as burnout. We are no longer productive. Ensuring we recognise the signs and symptoms is essential in detecting burnout early and may possibly help prevent burnout occurring in the first instance. *Where are you on this curve?*

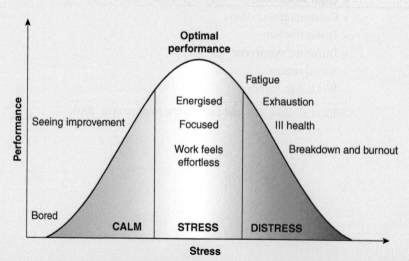

Stress, Evolution, and the Chimp

What happens to the brain when we immediately receive stressful news? For us to understand the internal processes of the brain, Steve Peters offers an excellent simplified view (Figure 1.2). In his seminal book *The Chimp Paradox*, Peters divides the brain into three parts. The 'chimp' represents the amygdala, the oldest part of the brain, which evolved purely to keep us safe and where the 'fight, flight, or freeze' response resides. It is an emotional and irrational part of the brain. The 'human', representing the frontal lobe, is the logical, problem-solving part of the brain concerned with thriving. Thirdly, the 'computer', representing the parietal lobe, is where our automatic programmes, beliefs, and experiences are created and can be viewed as our habits.

Whenever there is a stressor, the first port of call is our 'chimp' (the emotional brain) and then the 'human' (the thinking brain) secondly. This is known as the amygdala hijack. The 'chimp' was crucial in times we were escaping sabre-toothed tigers and was developed to be highly attuned to stress. These stressors now are no longer real threats to our physical safety. Instead, we face social media, fear of litigation, news that someone else in another part of the country is getting sued, a demanding patient, or an ambiguous call from the practice manager.

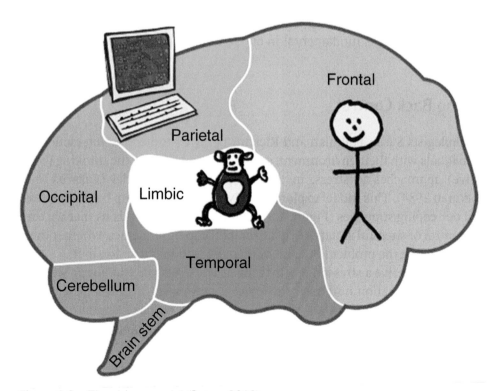

Figure 1.2 The chimp model (Peters 2012).

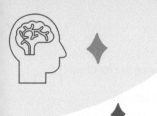

Think About It

- I avoid the situation.
- I criticise myself.
- I shut down and withdraw.
- I lash out.
- I turn to other activities to take my mind off things.
- I refuse to believe that it's happening to me.
- I use alcohol, drugs, or food to get me through it.
- I excessively worry about the worst case of the situation.
- I feel like I will not be able to cope.
- I make fun of the situation and turn to humour.
- I make a plan.

Without being aware of how to optimise to mind and bypass the 'chimp', using the 'computer' to create new positive habits, we are at the mercy of the increasing number of external triggers we are exposed to throughout our days as dental professionals. We run the risk of being solely driven by our 'chimp'. To build emotional resilience and real well-being, we need to be aware that mind training is fundamental in our abilities to flourish.

Taking Back Control

Psychologists Susan Folkman and Richard Lazarus studied the interaction of individuals with their environment, specifically considering the thinking (cognitive) approaches to stress, in their Coping Theory model (Lazarus and Folkman 1984). This model explores the dynamic relationship between stress and our coping strategies (Figure 1.3). Coping Theory reminds us that we can get control of stressful situations, using helpful coping strategies, whether they are focused on the problem in hand or on our emotional reaction to it.

When we receive a stressor, whether this is work related or at home, we first appraise the situation in terms of whether it may cause us harm, threat, or a challenge (primary appraisal). We then move onto a second appraisal where we assess if we can cope with the stressor. We do this by considering various coping options to best change the situation (coping response). Problem-focused coping attempts to change the stress by practical means. If this is not possible, emotion-focused coping aims to reduce our negative emotional state. Both

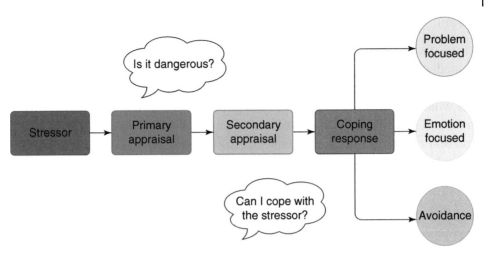

Figure 1.3   Coping theory (Lazarus and Folkman 1984).

problem- and emotion-focused coping styles are helpful, dependent on the situation. The third category of coping style is avoidance, and as the name suggests, it is unhelpful (in the long term)! See Figure 1.4 for examples for each coping style.

Problem-focused coping	**Emotion-focused coping**	**Avoidant thinking**
• Modify sources of stress directly • Make a plan for action • Improving time management • Analysing what you can take on • Talking to someone who can help change the situation	Positive: • Controlling your response to a stressor • Acceptance of responsibility • Positive reframing • Looking for learning/ growth • Social support • Mindfulness • Prayer • Journaling • Humour Negative: • Alcohol/drugs • Comfort eating • Brooding • Self-blame	• Avoid thinking by distractions/ entertainment • Denial

Figure 1.4   Coping responses to stress.

Chronic Stress: A Recipe for a Frazzled Brain

As we discussed in the previous section, our brain has evolved to manage an immediate response to imminent danger. As the Yerkes–Dodson Curve describes, a certain amount of stress can be helpful in making us feel energised. But what does chronic stress do to our brains? Neuroscience research of the brain and stress reveal that chronic stress physically changes the structure and function of our brain. The chronic stressors dental professionals face in the workplace dangerously deregulate a system built only to deal with short-term responses.

Key changes to the brain due to chronic stress:

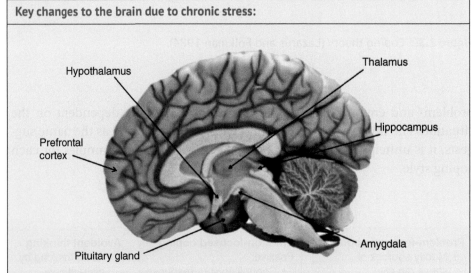

Source: Samata Behavioral Health and Wellness Institute, LLC.

- Pituitary gland stimulates the adrenal gland to release more cortisol.
- Cortisol causes hippocampus to shrink – reducing our ability to learn and remember.
- Pre-frontal cortex shrinks – reducing our concentration, decision-making, judgment, and social interaction abilities.
- Sensory cortex sends fear signals to the body, creating physical symptoms.
- Levels of dopamine and serotonin drop.
- Amygdala (aka 'chimp') becomes overactive.
- Protein BDNF (brain-derived neurotrophic factor) is slowed down – major contributor in the growth and maintenance of neural cells.
- Increases risk of depression and Alzheimer's disease.

Burnout and Compassion Fatigue

As with our other healthcare comrades, burnout and compassion fatigue are occupational hazards of the role. Both are risk factors for depression and anxiety, suicide, alcohol and drug misuse, patient errors, strained work relationships, patient dissatisfaction, and attrition (Lacy and Chan 2018).

Burnout is defined as chronic workplace stress where we are unable to meet constant demands (World Health Organization 2019) and is as high as 30% of dental clinicians (Toon et al. 2019). It often develops at undergraduate level and presents as a higher risk in dental students compared with other university students (Collin et al. 2020). Clinician burnout is problematic in severely impacting our well-being, professional efficacy, and ability to look after patients.

Burnout can be thought as a three-dimensional construct incorporating high emotional exhaustion, high depersonalisation and low levels of personal accomplishment' (Maslach and Jackson 1986). Depersonalisation refers to a reduced engagement with one's life; a psychological withdrawal from relationships and the development of a negative, cynical attitude. Dental professionals early on in their careers may be at increased susceptibility to depersonalisation and work–life conflicts. Research on medical professionals also highlights that traits of perfectionism and extreme dedication to providing exceptional care may compel healthcare professionals to prioritise professional duties disproportionately over time spent maintaining their own well-being. Emotional exhaustion refers to feeling very low in energy, a deep exhaustion not resolved with rest, and a reduced ability to feel empathy. As a dental professional, empathy is one of our prized values, and this greatly impacts our communication and ability to connect with our patients. Reduced personal accomplishment in the context of dentistry is the loss of feeling like the work you are doing is worthwhile and helps patients.

A simplified way to remember the signs and symptoms of burnout is to break down its impact on our thoughts, feelings, and actions (see Figure 1.5). The thoughts that characterise burnout are deep cynicism related to work and hopelessness and being self-critical in nature, such as 'what's the point in trying, I'm never good enough', 'I'm not a good dentist', 'my patients/co-workers don't care about the hard work I'm doing'. Dental professionals may feel incompetent, inefficient, and unable to complete tasks. The thoughts often present in a ruminative fashion, an endless loop of excessive worry and a decrease in focus. In terms of the emotional impact of burnout, there is a severe emotional exhaustion. Energy levels are grossly depleted, and burnt-out dental professionals feel a reduced ability to feel empathy. The latter is particularly critical when working within dentistry, as our ability to connect to our patients with compassion is diminished. And lastly, the impact of burnout on our behaviours includes taking time off (absenteeism), inability to work or be productive on days when we come into clinic (presenteeism), and leaning towards unhelpful coping strategies, such as substance abuse. We can see from Figure 1.5 that burnout impacts how we think, how we feel, and our actions. For this reason, it is imperative we value, understand and actively train the mind muscles of resilience.

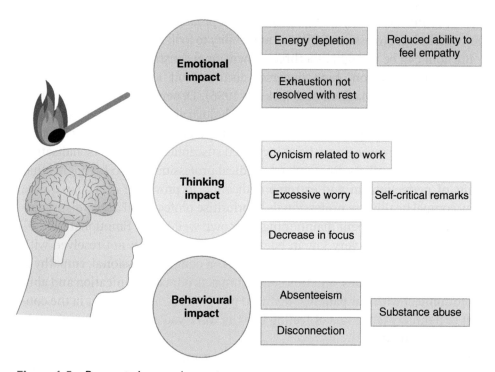

Figure 1.5 Burnout signs and symptoms.

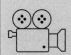

Learning From Movies

A Case Study: Meredith Grey from Grey's Anatomy

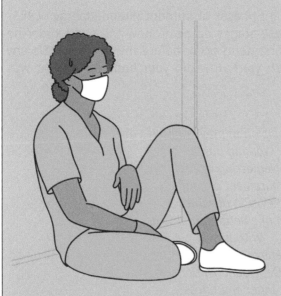

The character of Meredith Grey in the popular TV series *Grey's Anatomy* experiences multiple incidences of secondary trauma, from her husband dying to watching her mother's attempted suicide to removing a live bomb from a patient's body and watching it explode. Her burnout presents itself in Meredith's unstable behaviour: withdrawal, lack of interest, presenteeism, and energy depletion. Similarly to Meredith's character, working as a dental professional involves working closely with patients acutely experiencing all sorts of trauma, from a cancer diagnosis to mental health challenges. In addition, we manage complex treatment plans and balance our own well-being. Having these real experiences conveyed through pop culture is so important in beginning to identify burnout in ourselves. We can see a version of what that experience emotionally and physically looks like, and in many ways that can be more powerful than simply reading the signs and symptoms.

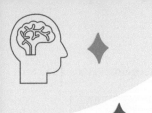

Think About It

H.J. Freudenberger describes 12 phases of burnout (Freudenberger 1986), outlined below. In reality these stages do not follow the exact order he described but generally the first items occur before the last items. Do any of these stages resonate with you? How did your body feel? What was happening emotionally?

Compulsion to prove oneself
Working harder
Neglecting needs
Displacement of conflicts
Revision of values
Denial of emerging problems
Withdrawal
Behavioural changes
Depersonalisation
Inner emptiness
Depression
Collapse

Measure Your Well-being: Burnout

Try the gauges below, rating your levels of the three subsections of burnout (emotional exhaustion, depersonalisation, and personal accomplishment) by answering the prompt below for each gauge (adapted from the Maslach Burnout Inventory Scale, 1981). A high score for emotional exhaustion and depersonalisation and a lower score on personal accomplishment may indicate burnout.

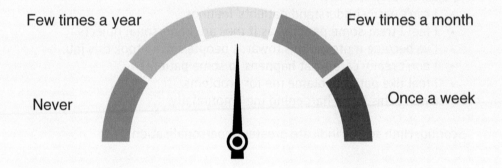

Once a month or less

Few times a year

Few times a month

Never

Once a week

Emotional exhaustion

How often do the following statements describe the way you feel working as a dental professional?
- I feel emotionally drained from work.
- I feel fatigued when I get up in the morning.
- Working with patients all day is really a strain for me.
- I feel frustrated by my job.

Scoring: High scores indicate greater emotional exhaustion.

Measure Your Well-being: Burnout

Once a month or less

Few times a year   Few times a month

Never   Once a week

Depersonalisation

How often do the following statements describe the way you feel working as a dental professional?
- I can't easily understand patients' feelings.
- I feel I treat some patients as if they are impersonal objects.
- I've become more callous towards people since I took this job.
- I don't really care what happens to some patients.
- I feel like patients blame me for problems.
- I worry this job is hardening me emotionally.

Scoring: High scores indicate greater depersonalisation.

Once a month or less

Few times a year   Few times a month

Never   Once a week

Personal accomplishment

How often do the following statements describe the way you feel working as a dental professional?
- I feel like I am positively influencing patients' lives through my work.
- I feel exhilarated after working closely with patients.
- I feel I can effectively deal with the problems of my patients.
- I have accomplished worthwhile things in my job.

Scoring: High scores indicate greater personal accomplishment.

Left unaddressed, clinician burnout may progress to the very serious syndrome known as compassion fatigue. Compassion fatigue is the emotional and physical burden of caring for patients in distress. It shares similar symptoms with post-traumatic stress disorder (PTSD). As dental professionals manage a range of patients with chronic illnesses, social struggles, mental health problems, and trauma, we are at risk of absorbing our patients' suffering. Special care and oral and maxillofacial surgery fields of dentistry in particular may be at an increased risk of compassion fatigue. Compassion fatigue in clinicians is defined as burnout with the addition of secondary trauma (see Figure 1.6); that is, feelings of distress and guilt when we are unable to do our best for our patients. An example of the latter includes the distress felt when we are unable to remove our paediatric patients' infected tooth due to patient anxiety and need to refer onto general anaesthetic services, where there is an incredibly long waiting list.

As with burnout, it is worth thinking of the signs of symptoms of compassion fatigue in relation to its impact on our emotions, thoughts, and behaviours (see Table 1.3).

The flip of clinician burnout and compassion fatigue is enhancing levels of work engagement. Work engagement is a positive construct, approaching working life with vigour, dedication, and absorption. To find out how we can boost our levels of work engagement, see Chapter 10, where we explore character strengths.

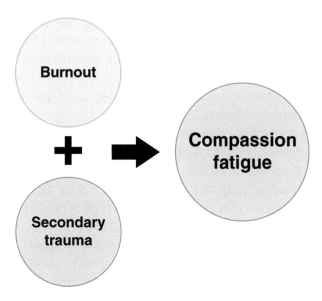

Figure 1.6   Compassion fatigue.

Table 1.3 Signs and symptoms of compassion fatigue.

Emotions	Thoughts	Behaviours
• Fearful and anxious • Hopelessness and sadness • Nightmares or flashbacks • Panic attacks • Loss of morale • Feelings of existential despair • Loss of self-worth and emotional modulation • Nervous system arousal (sleep disturbance)	• Increase in negative thoughts • Identity, worldview, and spirituality impacted • Cognitive ability decreases	• Alcohol/drug use • Withdrawal • Compulsive behaviours • Rechecking locks or checking personal safety

A Mental Health Crisis

Summary key research findings of mental health and well-being of dental professionals:

- Chronic work-related stressors translate to high costs to the health of dental professionals. High levels of stress are related to increased incidences of burnout (Rada and Johnson-Leong 2004; Alexander 2001). Ten percent of UK general dental professionals (GDPs) had thoughts of committing suicide, much higher than the general population of 5% (Toon et al. 2019).
- Burnout may start at undergraduate level; there are high burnout levels in dental students compared with the general population. Thirty-five percent of UK dental students exhibited increased levels of burnout, distress, maladaptive perfectionism, and infective coping strategies (Collin et al. 2020).
- Type A personality traits may put dentists at higher risk of burnout; for example, the archetypal personality with high scores in extroversion, sensing, thinking, and judging (Baran 2005).
- GDPs are at higher risk of anxiety compared with specialists, perhaps due to specialists having more control over their workload and more confidence in interacting with patients due to further training (Puriene et al. 2008).

- Strict professional regulation may be a factor in stress and burnout.
- Dentists are required to always act professionally and hide their emotions. This can result in a discrepancy between required and felt emotions, known as emotional dissonance, which in turn leads to emotional suppression (Chapman et al. 2015).
- Stigma inhibits professionals from seeking support (Rada and Johnson-Leong 2004).
- Impact on patients: anxiety and burnout may impact clinical decision-making and decision-making style (Chapman et al. 2017).

Recommendations for change:

- Curriculum changes: Psychological well-being training, including stress management, needs to be embedded into the dental curriculum and should include information about coping strategies, including maladaptive perfectionism and how to address this (Collin et al. 2020).
- Organisational changes: Interventions should target addressing stressors by making changes to the working conditions of dentists (Toon et al. 2019).

Breaking the Burnout Cycle

The causes of the mental health crisis in dentistry are multifactorial: from strict professional regulation causing a fear of litigation, organisational factors (admin, staffing issues, high targets) to clinical (difficult cases and patients) and individual factors (personality traits, stigma, imposter syndrome). The solutions, therefore, need to be multifaceted and holistic, with all groups pulling together.

The optimistic finding from research on interventions is that poor mental health outcomes may be preventable. Research on burnout prevention and optimising mental health in healthcare professionals points to psychological programmes (Kunzler et al. 2020). Mindfulness-based stress reduction (MBSR) interventions have been shown to enhance emotional awareness and reduce anxiety. Thinking and behavioural interventions (cognitive behavioural training) have demonstrated enhanced resilient thinking. Furthermore, evidence for the efficacy of resilience training in boosting well-being and decreasing burnout and depressive symptoms for healthcare professionals displays very promising results despite being in its infancy (Astin 1997; Shapiro et al. 1998; Teasdale et al. 2000; Goodman and Schorling 2012; Mache et al. 2016). Research in healthy and clinical populations shows that psychological resilience training reduces burnout, depression, and anxiety scores. One interesting study based their intervention on the Penn Resilience Programme (the flagship resilience training from Martin Seligman and Karen Reivich) reported increases in coping skills, resilience, and positive emotions amongst Chinese medical students (Peng et al. 2014).

Curriculum and organisational changes are crucial to address these issues on a wider scale. To read more on recommendations for change, see Chapter 13 for a comprehensive look at positive actions for dental teams and the wider dental healthcare system.

Spectrum of Interventions for Mental Health

Preventative Interventions

In the spectrum of interventions for mental health (see Figure 1.7), clinician psychological programmes, like the ones mentioned in the research, are classified as preventative for dental professionals who are well or with some mild symptoms. This book also falls into this preventative category.

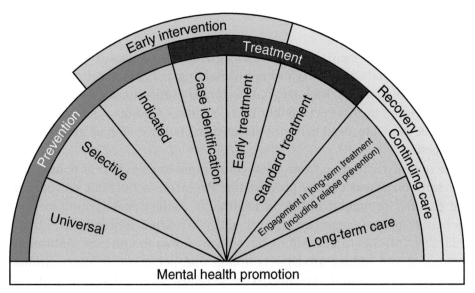

Figure 1.7 Spectrum of interventions for mental health. Adapted from Commonwealth Department of Health and Aged Care 2000.

Resilience and Well-being for Dental Professionals acts as your personalised mental well-being toolkit, encouraging you to integrate your own self-interventions through breaking down the evidence base into practical strategies to boost positive emotions, positive thoughts, and positive actions.

Another excellent preventative action comes from the Mental Health Wellness in Dentistry framework, which was introduced in June 2021. This is the first UK framework within the profession that highlights the need for stress awareness training and maintenance of skills for the dental team (see Mental Health Wellness in Dentistry Framework 2021). Dental teams, hospitals, and community practices are encouraged to appoint a mental well-being lead who is trained in mental health first aid and suicide awareness and encouraged to ensure that the team members are trained in stress management.

Further to these recommendations, it is my personal opinion that all dental team members should be trained in mental health first aid. In this way, the entire dental team learns how to spot early signs and symptoms of psychological distress in their colleagues and how to compassionately communicate with and support them. It also allows for every team member to help support each other. Additionally, annual resilience and well-being training must also be a priority for dental teams. Well-being is more than the absence of illness. And for this reason, our interventions should not only focus on reducing negative well-being markers but also help dental professionals feel happier, healthier, engaged at work, and thriving.

Early Interventions

Early interventions are targeted for professionals who are moving from mild mental health issues to mental illness. These may include visiting the GP, engaging in psychotherapy, and medication.

Treatment for Mental Illness

For a dental professional who is very unwell with a diagnosis of mental illness, a range of treatment and support approaches are available to assist in recovery, including engagement with longer-term treatment and care and relapse care prevention.

Summary

- We are all on the mental health continuum.
- Where we sit on the continuum depends upon our life circumstances, genes, risk factors, and protective factors.
- Protective factors for positive mental health include emotional regulation, self-awareness, mindfulness, thinking flexibility, meaning, positive relationships, community, nutrition, sleep, and exercise.
- Protective factors can enhance well-being.
- Burnout and compassion fatigue are occupational hazards of dentistry.
- Burnout is characterised by low personal accomplishment, high emotional exhaustion, and high depersonalisation.
- Occupational hazards may be preventable through a multifactorial positive approach taken by regulatory bodies, governing bodies, dental organisations, dental teams, education, and academia as well as individual approaches, such as integrating daily well-being activities.

 The View From Here

We put so much emphasis on training the muscles of our body, but have you ever thought about working out the most important muscle of them all – your mind? It was pretty revolutionary to me when I first delved into psychology that you can absolutely build the muscles of self-compassion, optimism, resilience, emotional intelligence, mindset, grit, and focus! There are numerous benefits of exercising the brain. We can bolster our protective factors even in response to life's adversities, reduce chronic stressors from piling up, and decrease our chances of developing burnout, compassion fatigue, and mental health problems. We can shift towards thriving – moving beyond baseline to optimal states, from boosting our happiness levels, meaning, and engagement at work to enhancing our life satisfaction.

The next chapters of this book provide you with the brain workout exercises, drawing upon evidence-based tools of positive psychology, neuroscience, and mindfulness, to support you in practically applying the research when with patients and at home. Ultimately, it is these intentional, small actions that can make all the difference to us feeling good.

References

Alexander, R.E. (2001). Stress-related suicide by dentists and other health care workers. Fact or folklore? *Journal of the American Dental Association (1939)* 132 (6): 786–794.

Astin, J. (1997). Stress-reduction through mindfulness meditation: effects on psychological symptomatology, sense of control, and spiritual experiences. Master's thesis. Submitted for publication.

Baran, R.B. (2005). Myers Briggs type indicator, burnout, and satisfaction in Illinois dentists. *General Dentistry* 53 (3): 228–235.

Chapman, H., Chipchase, S., and Bretherton, R. (2015). Understanding emotionally relevant situations in primary care dental practice: 1. Clinical situations and emotional responses. *British Dental Journal* 219: 401–409.

Chapman, H., Chipchase, S., and Bretherton, R. (2017). The evaluation of a continuing professional development package for primary care dentists designed to reduce stress, build resilience and improve clinical decision-making. *British Dental Journal* 223: 261–271.

Collin, V., Toon, M., O'Selmo, E. et al. (2019). A survey of stress, burnout and well-being in UK dentists. *British Dental Journal* 226: 40–49.

Collin, V., O'Selmo, E., and Whitehead, P. (2020). Stress, psychological distress, burnout and perfectionism in UK dental students. *British Dental Journal* 229: 605–614.

Commonwealth Department of Health and Aged Care (2000). *Promotion, Prevention and Early Intervention for Mental Health – A Monograph*. Canberra: Mental Health and Special Programs Branch, Commonwealth Department of Health and Aged Care.

Freudenberger, H.J. (1986). The issues of staff burnout in therapeutic communities. *Journal of Psychoactive Drugs* 18 (3): 247–251.

Goodman, M.J. and Schorling, J.B. (2012). A mindfulness course decreases burnout and improves well-being among healthcare providers. *International Journal of Psychiatry in Medicine* 43 (2): 119–128.

Kay, E.J. and Lowe, J.C. (2008). A survey of stress levels, self-perceived health and health-related behaviours of UK dental practitioners in 2005. *British Dental Journal* 204 (11): E19.

Kunzler, A.M., Helmreich, I., Chmitorz, A. et al. (2020). Psychological interventions to foster resilience in healthcare professionals. *Cochrane Database of Systematic Reviews* 7 (7): CD012527. https://doi.org/10.1002/14651858.CD012527.pub2.

Lacy, B.E. and Chan, J.L. (2018). Physician burnout: the hidden health care crisis. *Clinical Gastroenterology and Hepatology* 16 (3): 311–317.

Lazarus, R. and Folkman, S. (1984). *Stress, Appraisal, and Coping*. New York: Springer.

Mache, S., Bernburg, M., Baresi, L., and Groneberg, D.A. (2016). Evaluation of self-care skills training and solution-focused counselling for health professionals in psychiatric medicine: a pilot study. *International Journal of Psychiatry in Clinical Practice* 20 (4): 239–244.

Maslach, C. and Jackson, S.E. (1986). *Maslach Burnout Inventory Manual*, 2e. Palo Alto, CA: Consulting Psychologists Press.

Mental Health Wellness in Dentistry Framework (2021). www.mhwd.org (accessed 20 June 2021).

Newton, J.T., Baghaienaini, F., Goodwin, S.R. et al. (1994). Stress in dental school: a survey of students. *Dental Update* 21 (4): 162–164.

Newton, J.T., Allen, C.D., Coates, J. et al. (2006). How to reduce the stress of general dental practice: the need for research into the effectiveness of multifaceted interventions. *British Dental Journal* 200: 437–440.

Peng, L., Li, M., Zuo, X. et al. (2014). Application of the Pennsylvania resilience training program on medical students. *Personality and Individual Differences* 61–62: 47–51.

Peters, S. (2012). *The Chimp Paradox*. Vermilion.

Puriene, A., Aleksejuniene, J., Petrauskiene, J. et al. (2008). Self-perceived mental health and job satisfaction among Lithuanian dentists. *Industrial Health* 46 (3): 247–252.

Rada, R.E. and Johnson-Leong, C. (2004). Stress, burnout, anxiety and depression among dentists. *Journal of the American Dental Association* (1939) 135 (6): 788–794.

Shapiro, S.L., Schwartz, G.E., and Bonner, G. (1998). Effects of mindfulness-based stress reduction on medical and premedical students. *Journal of Behavioral Medicine* 21: 581–599.

Teasdale, J., Segal, Z.Y., Williams, M. et al. (2000). Prevention of relapse/recurrence in major depression by mindfulness-based cognitive therapy. *Journal of Consulting and Clinical Psychology* 68: 615–623.

Toon, M., Collin, V., Whitehead, P., and Reynolds, L. (2019). An analysis of stress and burnout in UK general dental practitioners: sub dimensions and causes. *British Dental Journal* 226: 125–130.

World Health Organization (2004). Promoting mental health: concepts, emerging evidence, practice (summary report).

World Health Organization (2019). *International Statistical Classification of Diseases and Related Health Problems*, 11e. Geneva, Switzerland: World Health Organization.

Yerkes, R.M. and Dodson, J.D. (1908). The relation of strength of stimulus to rapidity of habit-formation. *Journal of Comparative Neurology and Psychology* 18 (5): 459–482.

2

Applying the Science of Well-being

CHAPTER OVERVIEW

- Understanding what well-being means
- Measuring your well-being
- Understanding the building blocks of thriving: PERMA model
- PERMA plus
- Other theories of well-being
- Evidence on psychological interventions in dentistry and medicine.

Psychological well-being is more than the absence of depressive feelings and anxiety – it incorporates feeling good, optimistic, connected with others, and engaged with our lives and living a rich and meaningful life. As busy dental professionals, creating a career that is flourishing and a personal life that nourishes and inspires us, we could benefit enormously from unpacking the science of well-being. The research from positive psychology, the scientific study of what makes individuals and organisations thrive, has many applications to dental professionals. It incorporates happiness, self-compassion, emotional intelligence, mindset, motivation, strengths, positive communication, and meaning to resilience and post-traumatic growth. Since the conception of psychology study, there has been a sharp focus on the negative aspects of life that contribute to psychological health amongst the research rather than positive factors. Positive psychology addresses this imbalance. In this and subsequent chapters, we explore how we can use the research to improve our own well-being.

The Two Types of Well-being

Positive psychology draws some of its key principles from philosophy. Two different types of well-being explored in the literature are known as hedonic well-being and eudaimonic well-being. The origins of the two types date back to ancient Greek philosophers around 400 BCE: hedonism by Aristippus and eudaimonia by Aristotle. Hedonic well-being refers to happiness from feeling pleasure in the moment. The problem with this, however, is that it is fleeting, and we need to constantly top up our levels to maintain its effects. Eudaimonic well-being taps into happiness we gain from having meaning in our lives and aligning to a purpose that is bigger than ourselves. Although we do need pleas-

Satisfaction with life + positive emotion − negative emotion = well-being.

ure in our lives, the psychology research suggests that pursuing meaning is strongly related to happiness compared with just pursuing pleasure (Schueller and Seligman 2010).

Another way to think about well-being is considering how we evaluate our life and the interplay with our positive and negative emotion levels. This is known as subjective well-being. Subjective-well-being has three parts, one evaluative and the other two focused on our mood. In positive psychology, it is expressed as the following handy formula:

This translates as how we think about our life, in terms of our expectations and resemblance to our 'ideal' life, plus how positive we feel minus how negative we feel. See the *Measure Your Well-being* worksheet to measure your satisfaction with life and positive emotions.

Languishing versus Flourishing

Do you ever feel a bit disengaged? Like you are on a treadmill, just going through the motions but not really feeling engaged with your life? There is actually a term for this very common feeling: languishing. Coined as the neglected middle child of mental health by some, languishing describes the feeling of stagnation, feeling unsettled but not highly anxious and unmotivated. Moods may appear not too high or low. You may not feel happy, but you also do not feel sad. It is the gap between depression and flourishing – the absence of well-being.

Corey Keyes, a psychologist and socialist, was the first to describe both concepts in relation to mental well-being. Flourishing, otherwise known as thriving, refers to a state of mental wellness; we feel good, engaged, connected, fulfilled, and positively challenged. In the next section, we explore what the building blocks to thriving look like.

Measure Your Well-being

Measure your well-being using the Satisfaction with Life Scale (Diener et al. 1985), followed by the Positive and Negative Affect Schedule (PANAS) (Watson et al. 1988). You can then use your results to work out your subjective well-being score.

Satisfaction with Life Scale

Below are five statements that you may agree or disagree with. Using the 1–7 scale below, indicate your score for each statement. Try to be as open and honest in your scoring as possible.

7 – Strongly agree
6 – Agree
5 – Slightly agree
4 – Neither agree nor disagree
3 – Slightly disagree
2 – Disagree
1 – Strongly disagree

___ In most ways my life is close to my ideal.
___ The conditions of my life are excellent.
___ I am satisfied with my life.
___ So far I have gotten the important things I want in life.
___ If I could live my life over, I would change almost nothing.

Scoring: Add each item to get your Satisfaction with Life score. Below are suggested meanings for score ranges, according to the authors.

31–35 Extremely satisfied
26–30 Satisfied
21–25 Slightly satisfied
20 Neutral
15–19 Slightly dissatisfied
10–14 Dissatisfied
5–9 Extremely dissatisfied

Measure Your Well-being: Subjective Well-being

PANAS

For each item, indicate the extent you generally feel the different feelings and emotions, on average.

1 – Very slightly or not at all
2 – A little
3 – Moderately
4 – Quite a bit
5 – Extremely

Emotion/feeling	Your rating
Interested	
Distressed	
Excited	
Upset	
Strong	
Guilty	
Scared	
Hostile	
Enthusiastic	
Proud	
Irritable	
Alert	
Ashamed	
Inspired	
Nervous	
Determined	
Attentive	
Jittery	
Active	
Afraid	

Scoring: To score the positive emotions add up the scores for the items in red. Scores may range anywhere from 10 to 50. Higher scores represent higher levels of positive emotions. To score the negative emotions, add up the scores on items that are in blue. Scores may range anywhere from 10 to 50. Higher scores represent higher levels of negative mood.

Were you surprised by the result? If the outcome was not as high as you would like, what small steps can you take to boost your positive mood?

Building Blocks of Thriving

PERMA is a positive psychology model of well-being that describes five building blocks to flourishing: **P**ositive emotions, **E**ngagement, **R**elationships, **M**eaning, and **A**ccomplishment (Seligman 2011). Research has shown significant associations between PERMA pillars and physical health, job satisfaction, life satisfaction, and organisational engagement (Kern Aet al. 2015). Umucu et al. (2020) examined PERMA among a sample of 205 student veterans. The authors reported that the PERMA questionnaire could help researchers and practitioners better gauge well-being in student veterans. Increasing each ingredient of PERMA can increase our levels of well-being through working on fostering positive thoughts, feelings, and actions. Before we consider how, let us delve into each pillar.

Positive emotions: Increasing our diet of positive emotions, from optimism, curiosity, awe, and zest to compassion, looks different for every individual. As a community that emphasises productivity, this strand of PERMA is the focus on doing more activities that make you feel good. At work, this could be actively practicing gratitude during a morning team huddle, recalling positive moments with patients, practicing mindfulness for two minutes pre a team meeting or during your work day with your nurse, or journaling about the funny moments during your day.

Engagement: This pillar focuses on activities that help you feel more engaged with your life. There are several routes to increase our levels of engagement, at work, and at home. This can be through activities that help us get into the 'flow' state, otherwise known as 'in the zone'. These are activities in which we get completely absorbed and lose track of time. Another route to engagement is doubling down on our strengths. To learn more about strengths, see Chapter 10.

Relationships: As humans, we are wired to be connected with loved ones. This pillar concentrates on the positive relationships at work and at home that bring us joy and support. This pillar is particularly crucial as dental professionals work in a multidisciplinary setting amongst dental nurses, hygienists, reception staff, specialists, and community services. Positive, caring, and supportive interpersonal connections are essential to our well-being at any stage of our life (Diener and Seligman 2002).

Meaning: This pillar concentrates on ways we feel fulfilled by leaning into causes or a purpose bigger than ourselves. This can be by thinking of big or small ways we can serve the community, creating a charity fundraiser, or even sending a motivational text to a friend who is struggling. To learn more about meaning, see Chapter 4.

Accomplishment: The last pillar focuses on ways we can feel more accomplished. This could be through setting weekly, monthly, or yearly goals that align with our values and what matters the most. To learn more about goals, see Chapter 12.

Additional Theories of Well-being

There are a number of important theories of well-being that are useful when we are thinking about practical ways we can an boost our levels of well-being. Many of the psychological interventions in the research are based on the theories below.

Broaden and Build (Fredrickson 1998): This theory describes the mechanism in which positive emotions broaden our thinking and help us build personal resources, such as resilience. Resilient people have been found to use positive emotions as ways of coping during adversity, such as humour (Werner and Smith 1992; Wolin and Wolin 1993; Masten 1994), creative exploration (Cohler 1987), relaxation, and optimistic thinking (Murphy and Moriarty 1976; Anthony 1987).

Mindfulness to Meaning Theory (Garland et al. 2015): Mindfulness allows individuals to decentre from stress into a state of awareness, which encourages broadening attention to reappraise life circumstances. This reappraisal is then further enhanced when individuals savour positive features of their environment, motivating behaviour driven by values and meaning in life. To learn more about mindfulness, see Chapter 6.

Attention Restoration Theory (Kaplan and Kaplan 1989): This theory describes the mechanism in which spending time in nature restores our concentration, through practice of effortless attention, and being in an unthreatening natural environment reduces stress and improves physiological functions, for example, heartrate and blood pressure.

Flow Theory (Csikszentmihalyi 1990): Flow, otherwise known as 'getting in the zone', is the feeling of being completely immersed in an activity. We lose track of time. We get inherent meaning and pleasure from this activity. Research shows flow has many routes to enhancing our well-being, our engagement at work and performance.

Self-Determination Theory (Ryan and Deci 2000): The three psychological needs identified in Self-Determination Theory (connection, choice, and competence) have been shown in the literature to be cross-culturally valued (Sheldon and Houser-Marko 2001) and related to well-being (Reis et al. 2000;

Sheldon et al. 1996). Furthermore, there is tremendous support for this theory in relation to a whole range of diverse topics from healthcare, medical education, mindfulness, exercise, and development to digital health and coaching.

Strengths Theory: This describes how the use of our character strengths, that is, the positive parts of our personality that impact how we think, act, and feel (e.g. creativity, social intelligence, and leadership), can improve well-being and resilience and help us thrive at work. To learn more about character strengths, read Chapter 10.

Barriers to Well-being

Did you know that there are a number of psychological obstacles that prevent us from building greater well-being? In this section we explore 3 key challenges.

The negativity bias: You may have noticed that we remember the negative things more than the positive. The analogy of negative news being like Velcro and positive as Teflon is often used to describe this natural negativity bias. The bias is due to how our brains have evolved to be highly attuned for threats and danger. Our amygdala kept us safe from predators, such as sabre tooth tigers, so prioritises the dangers. However, in today's age, the threats are not external and more about our self-concept, for example, as a result of social compassion.

   We can counteract our natural negativity bias through several evidence-backed ways. Practicing gratitude, that is, counting our blessings and how they make us feel, is one powerful strategy. Another method is the process of looking for silver linings, known as benefit finding, to highlight potential upsides to even difficult or challenging times.

Social comparison: This refers to the comparison we make with our peers to determine how well be are doing in life. Social media has certainly influenced our perception of how our peers are living and our ideas around success. With filters on top of beautifully curated feeds highlighting the best bits, social comparison presents many challenges. Social comparison in the research has been shown to influence our well-being; even if our standard of living is relatively good, if it is lower than our peer group, our well-being levels decrease (Solnick and Hemenway 1998).

Hedonic treadmill: The concept of the hedonic treadmill explains the mechanism in which pleasurable activities, such as buying a new phone, lose their shiny new appeal very quickly. This is why despite having a salary raise, getting married, or succeeding at something, and an initial raise in our happiness levels, we return to our happiness set points. The potential upside, however, to this adaptation is that when we receive bad news, we will feel worse in the short or medium term but then will eventually return to our original happiness levels.

Brain Training

There is a lot of attention paid to negative emotions, and it often seems there are relatively few positive emotions. Traditionally the medical model of care is to fix problems reactively rather than amplifying the positive aspects of life proactively. This is where positive psychology shines.

In the following sections, we explore practical ways you can apply the science of well-being to your life and counteract some of the obstacles we discussed above. All the exercises are designed to elevate our positive emotions. Through intentional well-being exercises, like the ones below, our brain responds by releasing important feel-good hormones:

> **Dopamine:** Motivates us to take action and achieve our goals and desires
> **Oxytocin:** Helps us to create meaningful connections with others
> **Serotonin:** Balances our mood
> **Endorphins**: Helps to alleviate anxiety released in response to stress or pain.

Sonja Lyubomirsky, an American psychologist, one of the leading scientists on happiness, describes several evidence-based strategies to boost our happiness levels (Lyubomirsky 2010).

Giving Thanks

Gratitude is a practice that is scientifically proven to benefit our levels of positive emotions and our relationships and also pay it forward in terms of helping others. Seligman's online study had participants journal about three good things that happened to them and reported increases in well-being and a reduction in depressive scores that were maintained up to a six-month follow-up! Try the gratitude journaling exercise (*Growing Gratitude*) to start reaping the benefits of gratitude. You can also experiment with variations of this gratitude practice, such as sharing your three gratitude points with family during your evening meal, writing a gratitude letter and sharing it with a person you want to thank, or listing your gratitude points. Try this for a week at a time, though. Consistent practice of one activity can get repetitive and reduces its impact.

Developing Your Coping Strategies

When we are so focused on looking after patients, it can be very easy as dental professionals to not prioritise our own self-care. To fill your cup means to replenish your stores of emotional and physical energy. Try the *Filling Your Cup* drawing activity to explore your self-care cup.

Cultivating Optimism

This is the belief in a future that is hopeful and bright. Optimism in positive psychology involves learning to think flexibly and accurately. To learn more about optimism, see Chapter 3 and try the *Developing an Optimistic Future Using Best Possible Self* journaling exercise in Chapter 11. The *Cultivating Optimism* exercise details one creative way to build optimism.

Nurturing Social Relationships

As humans, we are wired for strong social connection. One aspect that distinguishes very happy people from everyone else is if they have positive social support from friends and loved ones (Diener and Seligman 2002). Our social relationships help us grow and feel supported, nourish us during adversities, and even impact our physical health. Psychologist Dr. John Gottman's Sound House Relationship Theory provides an excellent framework for resilient relationships. The seven levels to the house are detailed below (Gottman and Gottman 2008):

1) **Building love maps:** The first level of the house is learning more about each other and regularly updating our knowledge of our partner or loved one. This involves staying curious and continuing to ask question about the other's psychological world –worries, stresses, joys, and dreams. Try the *Building Your Love Maps* worksheet to strengthen your romantic relationships.
2) **Sharing affection:** This focuses on cultivating affection and respect within a relationship. We can do this through expressing gratitude.
3) **Turning towards:** This means turning towards small bids of attention, that is, the small moments for positive connection – conversation, humour, affection, or support. These small bids of attention are opportunities to build relationship resilience. We can do this through being aware of each other's bids and turning towards them.
4) **Cultivating a positive perspective:** This is how we feel in the relationship. We can do this by using positive emotions during problem solving or revisiting positive memories. Another method is through the way we communicate

good news in our relationship (see section on Shelly Gable in Chapter 10). Gottman suggests a ratio of five positive interactions to one negative is important in creating strong, happy, and thriving relationships.

5) **Managing conflict:** Conflict in relationships is natural and has function. Positive aspects, for example, helping us better understand our partner better, deal with change and renew courtship over time. We can do this through buffering common communication negaters, such as contempt, stonewalling, criticism, and defensiveness.

6) **Making life dreams come true:** Making life dreams come true means creating a culture that encourages each person to talk honestly about dreams, values, aspirations, and what matters the most. This could involve helping your partner set goals aligning with values.

7) **Creating shared meaning:** This is what you tell yourself about your relationship and your internal thoughts, metaphors, and stories. We can encourage positive shared meaning stories though creating rituals of connection or supporting each other's life roles.

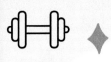

Growing Gratitude

1. Reflect on what you are grateful for over the last month. This could be accomplishments, things in progress, positive relationships, personal strengths, or personal growth. Write this down below.

2. How has this gratitude point benefited you and helped you develop? What would life look like without this?

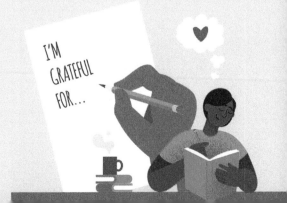

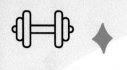

Growing Gratitude

3. Reflect on a gratitude moment at work, with a patient, a procedure that went well, or a colleague you are grateful for.

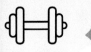

Filling Your Cup

1. Reflect on activities you enjoy that nourish you and help you feel taken care of. This could be taking a warm bath, reading, mindfulness, painting, running, or journaling.
2. Draw a cup in the space below.
3. Divide this cup into segments.
4. Fill each compartment with a drawing of a self-care activity. Use colouring pencils or paint to colour your drawings.
5. Keep your 'self-care cup' in a visible space to act as a visual reminder to schedule in 'me' time. Whenever you have a moment of spare time – this could be a minute or 5 – try one of your self-care activities. If you have any habits that you'd like to reduce, such as checking social media, you could instead try out your self-care ideas. In this way, you can ensure you have regular moments of time dedicated to yourself, throughout your day.

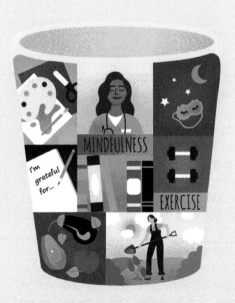

Here's an example of what your cup could look like.

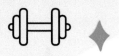

Cultivating Optimism

Visualising your future is a powerful tool in boosting levels of positive emotions, such as optimism. Visualisation can also be an effective way to keep goals top of mind. Athletes often use this technique when preparing for success. Try this vision board exercise and get your creative juices flowing.

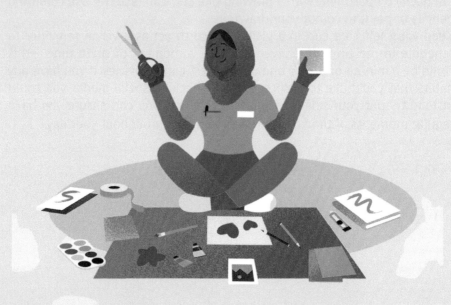

1. Reflect on your vision for your life in the next 6 months to a year. What do you want it to look like? You could think about personal growth, hobbies, career, relationships, or travel.
2. Use magazines or the internet as sources of inspiration. Source images and text that resonate with you.
3. Mindfully create a collage by cutting out images and words and placing them onto A3 paper or a board. Minimise distractions. Slow down and savour the process. Notice the sensation of pressing down the images onto your paper. Alternatively use apps, such as Canva, to create a digital vision board.
4. What are you most looking forward to doing from your board?
5. Place your vision board in a visible spot in your room. Alternatively, if you created a digital vision board, use it as your screensaver. Refer to your vision board during your day. Each time you look at it, imagine this future coming to life. How are you feeling?

Build Your Love Maps

Try the questions below with your romantic partner to help strengthen your love maps.

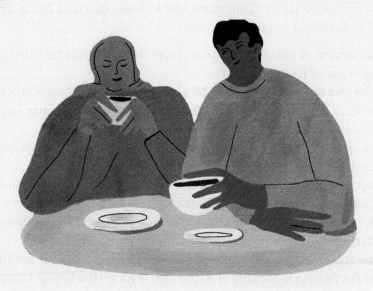

- Describe something that's exciting in your life right now.
- If you could instantly attain 3 skills, what would they be?
- What's the craziest thing you've ever done and would you do it again?
- What book has had the greatest impact on your life?
- What's your biggest fear for this relationship?
- Tell me something that you believed as a child that makes you laugh now.
- What's one of your favourite childhood memories?
- When was the last time a scent reminded you of a childhood memory? Share that story.
- Describe how you would spend a perfect Sunday.
- Which trip changed your life for the better?
- What do you know about life that few others have figured out yet?
- What choice had the greatest impact on your life?
- What's the best mistake you've ever made and why?
- What decision are you grateful you didn't make?
- Describe an argument you had that helped to shape the person you are today.
- Where in your life do you feel misunderstood?
- If you could time travel to an earlier time in your life, where would you visit and what would you do?
- What seemingly insignificant thing contributes greatly to your happiness?

Forgiving Others

Forgiveness can feel like an incredibly challenging and difficult decision, but holding resentment can cause us more suffering. There are multiple reasons why we do not forgive; we believe that forgiveness will empower the other person or subconsciously believe it to be a sign of weakness. However, it is impossible to go through life without another person hurting us. Forgiveness can be a very necessary and important tool to boost our well-being. Here are some tips to develop a forgiver's mindset:

- **Become aware of your inner pain:** Have the self-awareness that you are carrying anger or feelings of hurt.
- **Show forgiveness to yourself:** The ability to forgive others starts with us being able to forgive ourselves. Self-compassion is particularly important here. To learn more about self-compassion, read Chapter 7.
- **Make a commitment to do no harm:** Try to refrain from talking negatively about others.
- **Develop empathy:** Acknowledge that we all make mistakes and that's what connects us all. Try to put yourself in the other person's shoes. Consider that person's perspective. You may recognise that although you are suffering, the other person may also be in pain.
- **Find meaning in your suffering:** This is known as 'benefit finding' and involves the process of looking at adversities through the lens of reflection of life pre and post the adversity and our growth.
- **Call upon your values and strengths:** Reflect on your values, such as kindness, equality, inclusivity, and love, and use strengths such as courage to navigate the challenge.

Summary

- There are two types of well-being: hedonic well-being is related to pleasure and eudiamonic refers to happiness with meaning.
- Pursuing pleasurable activities feels great, but the value we get from creating a meaningful life is longer lasting.
- Languishing describes the feeling of stagnation, demotivation, and feeling unsettled.
- Flourishing is the opposite of languishing.
- PERMA describes five routes to flourishing: positive emotions, engagement, relationships, meaning, and accomplishment.
- Well-being interventions in medics show increases in well-being and decreases in negative well-being markers, such as burnout, anxiety, and depression.

- Practical ways to boost well-being include savouring using gratitude, developing coping strategies, optimism using the *Best Possible Self* exercise, nurturing social relationships, and forgiving others.
- It is important to find well-being activities that fit your personality and interests.
- Add variety to your routine by trying different well-being practices.

 ## The View From Here

Well-being is more than the absence of disease, and it is far from the packaged wellness from spa services and luxury holidays. Real well-being incorporates understanding who we are, our values, living a meaningful life, physical wellness, and feeling connected with loved ones. We can actively strengthen our well-being muscles through practising evidence-based strategies from positive psychology. Whether it is gratitude, mindfulness, random acts of kindness, mindful movement, or good sleep and nutrition, positive well-being requires intentional activities. In the subsequent chapters, we will inquire deeper into these well-being strategies. Although there is not a one-size-fits-all approach to boosting well-being, treat it more like an experiment. And the more experiments you make, the better!

References

Anthony, E.J. (1987). Risk, vulnerability, and resilience: an overview. In: *The Invulnerable Child* (ed. E.J. Anthony and B.J. Cohler), 3–48. New York: Guilford.

Cohler, B.J. (1987). Adversity, resilience, and the study of lives. In: *The Invulnerable Child* (ed. E.J. Anthony and B.J. Cohler), 363–424. New York: Guilford.

Csikszentmihalyi, M. (1990). *Flow: The Psychology of Optimal Experience.* New York: Harper & Collins.

Diener, E. and Seligman, M. (2002). Very happy people. *Psychological Science* 13 (1): 81–84.

Diener, E., Emmons, R.A., Larsen, R.J., and Griffin, S. (1985). The Satisfaction with Life Scale. *Journal of Personality Assessment* 49: 71–75.

Fredrickson, B.L. (1998). What good are positive emotions? *Review of General Psychology* 2 (3): 300–319.

Garland, E.L., Farb, N.A., Goldin, P.R., and Fredrickson, B.L. (2015). The mindfulness-to-meaning theory: extensions, applications, and challenges at the attention–appraisal–emotion interface. *Psychological Inquiry* 26 (4): 377–387.

Gottman, J.M. and Gottman, J.S. (2008). *Gottman method couple therapy. In Clinical Handbook of Couple Therapy* (ed. A.S. Gurman), 138–164. Guilford Press.

Kaplan, R. and Kaplan, S. (1989). *The Experience of Nature: A Psychological Perspective*. New York: Cambridge University Press.

Kern, M., Waters, L., Adler, A., and White, M. (2015). A multidimensional approach to measuring well-being in students: application of the PERMA framework. *Journal of Positive Psychology* 10: 262–271.

Lyubomirsky, S. (2010). *The How of Happiness*. Piatkus Books.

Masten, A.S. (1994). Resilience in individual development: successful adaptation despite risk and adversity. In: *Educational Resilience in Inner-City America: Challenges and Prospects* (ed. M.C. Wang and E.W. Gordon), 3–25. Hillsdale, NJ: Erlbaum.

Murphy, L.B. and Moriarty, A. (1976). *Vulnerability, Coping, and Growth: From Infancy to Adolescence*. New Haven, CT: Yale University Press.

Reis, H.T., Collins, W.A., and Berscheid, E. (2000). The relationship context of human behavior and development. *Psychological Bulletin* 126 (6): 844.

Ryan, R.M. and Deci, E.L. (2000). Self-determination theory and the facilitation of intrinsic motivation, social development, and well-being. *American Psychologist* 55 (1): 68–78.

Schueller, S. and Seligman, M. (2010). Pursuit of pleasure, engagement and meaning: relationships to subjective and objective measures of well-being. *Journal of Positive Psychology* 5 (4): 253–263.

Seligman, M.E.P. (2011). *Flourish: A Visionary New Understanding of Happiness and Well-being*. Free Press.

Sheldon, K.M. and Houser-Marko, L. (2001). Self-concordance, goal attainment, and the pursuit of happiness: can there be an upward spiral? *Journal of Personality and Social Psychology* 80 (1): 152–165.

Sheldon, K.M., Ryan, R., and Reis, H.T. (1996). What makes a good day? Competence and autonomy in the day and in the person. *Personality and Social Psychology Bulletin* 22: 1270–1279.

Solnick, S. and Hemenway, D. (1998). Is more always better? A survey on positional concerns. *Journal of Economic Behaviour and Organisation* 37: 373–383.

Umucu, E., Wu, J.R., Sanchez, J. et al. (2020). Psychometric validation of the PERMA-profiler as a well-being measure for student veterans. *Journal of American College Health* 68 (3): 271–277.

Watson, D., Clark, L.A., and Tellegen, A. (1988). Development and validation of brief measures of positive and negative affect: the PANAS scales. *Journal of Personality and Social Psychology* 54: 1063–1070.

Werner, E. and Smith, R. (1992). *Overcoming the Odds: High-risk Children from Birth to Adulthood*. New York: Cornell University Press.

Wolin, S.J. and Wolin, S. (1993). *Bound and Determined: Growing Up Resilient in a Troubled Family*. New York: Villard.

3

Rising with Resilience

CHAPTER OVERVIEW

- Understanding what resilience is
- Benefits of resilience
- Resilience research
- Post-traumatic growth
- Resilience protective factors
- Introducing the PERLE Resilience Model for Dental Professionals.

> *Resilience is not all or nothing. It comes in amounts. You can be a little resilient, a lot resilient; resilient in some situations but not in others. And, no matter how resilient you are today, you can become more resilient tomorrow.*
> —Karen Reivich, psychologist, professor at the University of Pennsylvania, and director for the Penn Resilience Program

What comes to mind when you think of the word 'resilience'? What qualities and strengths do resilient people you know possess? How about resilient teams?

Resilience is an essential tool for dental professionals navigating challenges and constant changes in the dental world. Furthermore, it is a critical life skill. Training our minds to become more resilient is essentially about learning how to tap into psychological tools to navigate adversities, recover, and grow through them. Far from the outdated 'bounce back' analogy, resilience actually is a journey, one that is dynamic, and there is no instant recoil back to recovery but a more compassionate finding of our internal resources and seeking social support.

The 'Tree of Life', located on the US West coast in Olympic National Park, Washington, has forged roots that supply the tree despite not having soil. This tree and countless others show nature's ability to adapt to different weather conditions; to bend with it rather than break. Similarly, resilience requires us to think flexibly, to roll with the rough and smooth. This dynamic process involves an interplay of protective factors in an individual, family,

Resilience and Well-being for Dental Professionals, First Edition. Mahrukh Khwaja.
© 2023 John Wiley & Sons Ltd. Published 2023 by John Wiley & Sons Ltd.
Companion website: www.wiley.com/go/khwaja-resilience-dentistry

peer network, and community that allows us to develop, maintain, and regain mental health despite adversity.

A great dental analogy of thinking about resilience is composite. It gains its strength by small increments of material that are cured. We can also gain mental strength by building ourselves up, one increment at a time. Similarly, team resilience can be thought as the capacity for a group of individuals to respond to change and adversities in an adaptive way. As dental professionals working in teams, safeguarding our team members through resilience and well-being training has tremendous benefits:

- Greater ability to regulate emotions
- Enhanced ability to handle challenges and stress
- Reduced occupational hazards, such as burnout and compassion fatigue
- Reduced presenteeism and absenteeism
- Enhanced communication
- Improved interpersonal relationships
- Openness in upskilling and developing
- Greater ability to give and receive support
- Increased authenticity at work.

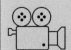 **Learning From Movies**

Disney's *Mulan* brings to life the Chinese legend of Hua Mulan, a female ancient Chinese warrior. It explores the theme of resilience through its protagonist. Mulan overcomes adversities she faces, both physically and psychologically. As seen through her experience of the army, Mulan hides her identity to protect her father by going in his place. We learn from this character that resilience requires a turning inwards to our internal psychological resources, such as optimism, self-awareness, and thinking flexibly, in addition to seeking support from allies. In the case of Mulan, it's the characters of Shang, Mushu, Ling, Chien-Po, and Yao who help Mulan at multiple points throughout the story. Similarly, as dental professionals we can help boost our resilience levels by seeking support from mentors, coaches, positive organisations, and friends.

Resilience Myths Debunked

Myth 1: Resilience Is Something You Either Have or Do Not

This is the most common myth surrounding resilience. And for many years, we believed that individuals possessed a fixed amount of resilience. We now know otherwise. Our brains have a special capacity to change structurally through experiences, known as neuroplasticity. With effort, new neural pathways for positive habits can be created at any age. Just as Karen Reivich emphasises in the quote at the start of this chapter, resilience indeed can be strengthened because, just like any muscle of the body, it can be trained. Without use, this muscle atrophies, and so continual active effort in mind training is essential.

Myth 2: Resilient People Do Not Have Problems or Stress

Being resilient does not mean you are immune to challenges. As we discussed in Chapter 1, in actuality, we are all on the mental health continuum. Our position on the continuum is influenced by what is going on in our lives. This means that any of us can shift into poorer mental health and lower resilience depending on negative life events. Resilient people buffer against these stressors by enhancing their well-being protective factors, hence actively building the muscle of resilience and minimising the risk of developing mental illness.

Myth 3: Resilient People Do Not Need Help

Resilience does not mean we are completely self-sufficient. Resilient people appreciate the importance of strong, positive relationships and community. When they experience adversities, they are comfortable in asking for help from others. This help could be from partners, friends, organisations, or professionals. Having loving, supportive relationships helps resilient people buffer against stressors, big or small.

Training the Brain for Greater Resilience

Unlike traditional psychology, which concentrates solely on what is wrong with an individual and how to fix it, positive psychology encourages individuals to recognise what is going right and amplify the positive. Evidence-based tools to build resilience and well-being come from this beautiful specialty of psychology. Interestingly, positive psychology already underpins positive education within schools, organisations, sports, and coaching and has started to make its way to healthcare, most notably with medical students.

Well-being Interventions

We are currently in a new era of increasing interest in psychological interventions targeted at strengthening well-being. To date, however, there are limited research studies that have examined interventions specifically targeting dental professionals. In this section, we explore the insight from these small studies. Cognitive-behavioural therapy (CBT) is explored later in this chapter, and mindfulness-based interventions are explored in Chapter 6.

In the last two decades, there have been three small counselling studies for postgraduate dental professionals (Newton et al. 2006; Gorter et al. 2000; Gònzalez and Quezada 2016) and three studies assessing the efficacy of CBT to enhance well-being (Chapman et al. 2017; Aboalshamat et al. 2015; Metz et al. 2020). Two of these studies targeted undergraduates and the third focused on GDPs. Encouragingly, all reported significant improvements in mental well-being, but these findings were limited due to use of different outcome measures and small selective sample sizes.

The literature for healthcare professionals, specifically our medical colleagues, is growing rapidly. Since medical professionals are most similar to dental professionals with regards to medical training, high stressors working closely with patients, long hours, and litigation, we can glean insights that could help to shape future interventions for dental professionals. The UK General Dental Council (GDC) recently recommended interventions to be adapted from other healthcare professions (Plessas et al. 2021). They argued that this should be part of contemporary education, both at the undergraduate and postgraduate level. Below we highlight some of the key intervention studies from other medical professions.

Medical Professionals

The research on interventions for medical professionals incorporates either predominantly or in combination CBT, mindfulness-based, positive psychology–based, support groups (known as Balint groups), or stress management. Sood et al. 2011 reported benefits of significant increase in resilience, decrease in perceived stress and anxiety, and increase in quality of life postintervention after a 90-minute Stress Management and Resilience Training (SMART), followed by 30–60 follow-up session. The SMART training included areas of positive psychology: attention, gratitude, compassion, acceptance, meaning, and forgiveness and components of mindfulness-based stress reduction (MBSR). The results of positive psychology interventions (PPIs), like this one, may be because of helping clinicians to enhance positive emotions despite adversities, such as the humble yet important emotions of gratitude, optimism, and compassion, and to leverage their values and character strengths to live a meaningful, engaged life and bring the best of them to patient interactions.

Although support groups are helpful in making us feel less isolated, they may be less effective than some other modalities. Four Balint groups reported by Clough et al. (2017) showed no evidence in enhancing well-being measures. Perhaps they were ineffective in stress and burnout prevention, as Balint groups do not target underlying thoughts associated with stress, enhance self-awareness or emotional regulation, or aid in coping skills that are necessary in building resilience. The equivalent of Balint groups in dentistry is study groups and local dental committee groups. Although they do provide a sense of community, they may be expensive to run and difficult to recruit consistent dental professionals to attend.

Medical Students

Dental students have very similar undergraduate training to medical students, not just in terms of curriculum but also with treating patients and having the responsibility of clinical care early on in their undergraduate training. Embedding resilience and well-being training into the dental undergraduate curriculum could be beneficial in teaching students the necessary mind tools early on in their careers and preventing subsequent burnout and poor mental health. Approaches that worked with the existing dental curriculum to enhance it with an emphasis on increasing students' protective factors for resilience – for example, incorporating virtues training highlighting benefits to both the clinician and patient – during communication sessions could be one method of bypassing the resistance from dental deans. Future research could also explore whether customised interventions would be possible, with autonomy for choosing different resilience elements, as these interventions are not a one size fits all. Additionally, dental student informed well-being components would be extremely beneficial in ensuring that the intervention is tailored to the needs of the cohort.

PPIs targeting medical students include mindfulness-based interventions (Rosenzweig et al. 2003) and character strengths as well as generalised positive psychology–based programmes (Machado et al. 2019) and the Penn Resilience Program (Peng et al. 2014). The Penn Resilience Program for a Chinese medical student cohort reported encouraging results (Peng et al. 2014). Resilience, positive emotions, and the cognitive appraisal scores of a low-resilience experimental group increased significantly after training. The positive results may be due to protective resilience factors – such as resilient thinking, positive emotions, leveraging character strengths, and nurturing positive relationships – being enhanced through this PPI. This study is limited, however, by no long-term follow-up and whether the positive results can be extrapolated to other cultures.

You 2.0

Another fascinating area in the research in resilience is the phenomenon known as post-traumatic growth (PTG). This describes the process in which individuals experience trauma, become further strengthened by it, reconfigure, and grow with capabilities greater than those preceding it. They become a 2.0 version of themselves! These individuals experience a positive growth as a result of their trauma. PTG does not deny the deep psychological distress; rather it recognises that positive psychological change may occur after a life crisis.

Resilience Protective Factors

In Chapter 1 we spotlighted the significance of protective factors on our levels of resilience and positive health. In this section we delve into these factors further. Let us take the analogy of an umbrella, imagining each spoke of this umbrella as an element of protection from life's invariable adversities (see Figure 3.1). The different spokes are explored below, summarising the key research findings on protective factors for greater resilience.

Genetics: Our biology plays a part in how resilient we naturally are. However, since this is the only factor we cannot directly influence, it is worth not being too hung up on your starting point.

Self-awareness: That is the awareness of our thoughts and emotions at any given moment. We are often more aware of our physical reaction to stress but less aware of our thoughts due to a disconnection between the mind and body.

Self-regulation: Once we are self-aware, we are then able to self-regulate, another key protective factor. This is the mind skill in recognising which thoughts or emotions may be helping or hindering us and finding strategies to influence those thoughts and calm our physiology when our brain is in a threat response (fight or flight mode).

Positive emotions: This includes the elevated emotions of love and happiness, not to discount the underrated yet humble emotions of gratitude, optimism, self-compassion, and curiosity.

Self-belief: Our ability to complete goals and master our environment, known as self-efficacy, is another crucial component. This impacts our choices, goal setting, effort, and persistence. We know that individuals with more self-efficacy are more likely to achieve difficult goals and try again despite rejections.

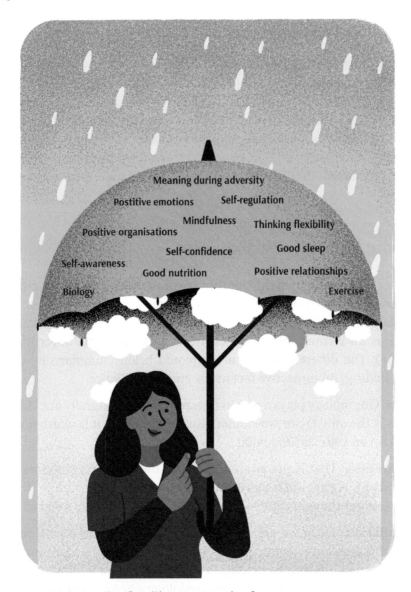

Figure 3.1   The umbrella of resilience protective factors.

Positive relationships and organisations: Since humans are hardwired for social connection, it is unsurprising that our community also provides us protection from adversities. Nurturing positive relationships and positive organisations is essential in building both resilience and our well-being.

Meaning: Essentially, meaning making despite pandemics or tragedies is centred in engaging in something bigger than ourselves. We may find meaning through spirituality or reflection. Research validates a strong correlation

Measure Your Well-being: Resilience

How resilient are you? Measure your current level of resilience using the brief resilience scale below (adapted from Smith et al. 2008).

For each statement, indicate the response that best applies to you, using the following scale.

Strongly disagree		Neutral		Strongly agree
1	2	3	4	5

___1. I tend to bounce back quickly after hard times.

___2. I have a hard time making it through stressful events.

___3. It does not take me long to recover from a stressful event.

___4. It is hard for me to snap back when something wrong happens.

___5. I usually come through difficult times with little trouble.

___6. I tend to take a long time to get over setbacks in my life.

Scoring:
First reverse the scores of items 2, 4, and 6. Reversing a score is done by exchanging the original value of an item by its opposite value; for example, a score of 1 turns into a score of 5, a score of 2 turns into a 4, and so forth. Add up all of the individual item scores and then divide by 6. Higher score indicates greater resilience levels.

between meaning and resilience. Interestingly, higher levels of meaning are also strongly correlated with better mental health, self-esteem, self-acceptance, and emotional regulation and a lower risk for substance abuse and addiction.

PERLE Resilience Model for Dental Professionals

Drawing from the research on the protective factors for resilience, PERMA, and lifestyle medicine, I present a resilience framework designed specifically for dental professionals: PERLE (see Figure 3.2). The PERLE Resilience Model for Dental Professionals describes five key pillars of building resilience at work: **P**urpose, **E**motional intelligence (divided into self-awareness, emotional regulation, and positive emotions), **R**esilient mindset, **L**ifestyle, and **E**nvironment at work (divided into High-Quality Connections [HQCs] and engagement). Increasing any pillar individually can increase our levels of psychological resilience and shift us towards engagement and thriving.

The analogy of the oyster and the pearl beautifully captures the process of resilience. When a grain of sand or another organism floats into the deepest parts of an oyster, the oyster begins to coat the foreign body and protect itself from the stressor, covering the painful intruder with layer upon layer of nacre. This makes up the oyster's inner shell. Over several years, these many layers create the beautiful, iridescent pearl. In the same way that the oyster uses its own internal resources to navigate stress and thrive, we can also use our own internal and external psychological resources when we face challenges in dentistry.

The PERLE model is designed to be used at the individual level, through supporting dental professionals in taking a proactive role in identifying areas they are lacking or wanting to strengthen and taking positive step forwards towards thriving. PERLE can also be used at the organisation level, with teams playing a critical role in building positive environments and dental organisations integrating the framework as part of resilience and well-being workshops and programmes.

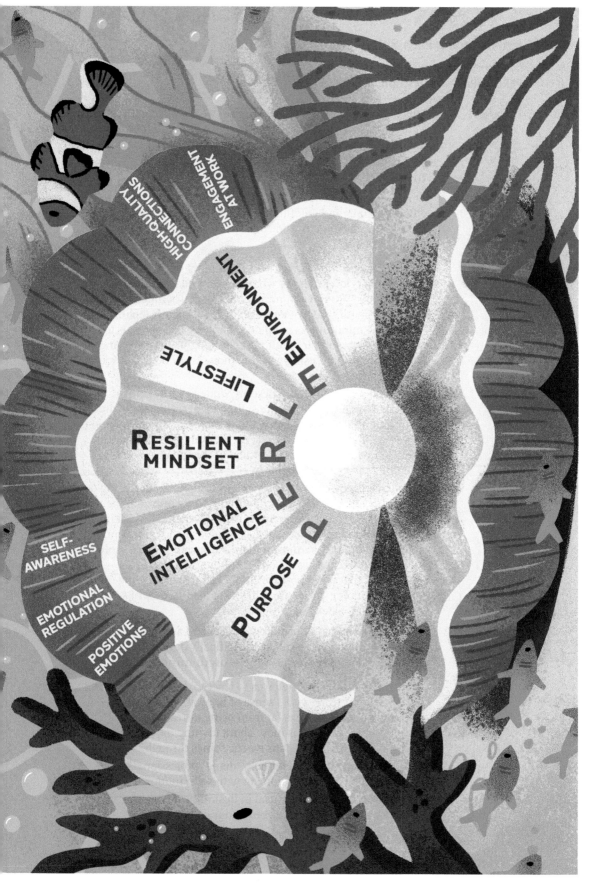

Figure 3.2 The PERLE framework.

Understanding Each Pillar

PERLE pillar	Description
Purpose	This pillar explores having meaning at work and alignment with a greater purpose than ourselves. This includes understanding our core values as dental professionals and creating goals that align with them. To learn more, see Chapter 4.
Emotional intelligence	Emotional intelligence (EI) is the ability to monitor our own and others' feelings and emotions, to discriminate among them and use this information to guide our own thinking and actions. This pillar splits into three sections: • **Self-awareness:** The first step in building greater emotional resilience is awareness of what we are thinking and feeling. We can do this through a mindful check-in, journaling, or taking a quiet moment to ask ourselves how are we really feeling right now. The mindfulness meditation process also helps us to become aware of our emotions and thoughts, by observing them rather than fusing with the thoughts or being sucked into the narrative of their stories. • **Emotional regulation:** These are strategies that help us regulate our negative emotions. Emotional regulation includes thinking strategies that help us to reframe events and situations in a way that is more helpful to us, for example, mindfulness, self-compassion, and CBT. The ability to regulate emotions is central to resilience building. • **Positive emotions:** As described in Chapter 2, increasing our diet of positive emotions is important in not only making us feeling good but also in helping us to broaden our thinking and build internal resources, such as resilience and optimism, physical strength, cardiovascular health, and problem-solving skills, and facilitating the quality of our relationships. Activities that boost positive emotions include spotting gratitude, going on nature walks, and using words of self-compassion instead of self-criticism.
Resilient mindset	Thinking styles that impact how we feel and act and are highly relevant to dental professionals, specifically developing **optimistic, compassionate,** and **growth mindsets.** • **Optimistic mindset** helps us to react to dental stressors and challenges at work with a sense of hope about the future. An optimistic perspective is far from being unrealistic and discounting reality; it is more about inviting more positivity through modifying the lens we see things through. • **Compassionate mindset** helps dental professionals replace self-criticism and perfectionism with self-kindness. • A **growth mindset** is crucial in upskilling as a dental professional and getting us out of our comfort zones. See Chapters 7 and 8 for a focus on resilient mindsets.

PERLE pillar	Description
Lifestyle	This pillar recognises the impact of our physical health, particularly sleep, movement, and nutrition, on our psychological well-being. See Chapter 9 for an in-depth look at lifestyle factors.
Environment at work	This pillar focuses on cultures at work that are kind, compassionate, and positive. It is split into two parts:

- **High-Quality Connections (HQCs):** HQCs acknowledge the importance of positive relationships at work in building resilience. HQCs can be micro-moments of connection that work to increase our resilience through increasing our levels of positive emotions. We can do this through prioritising mindful interactions with our colleagues, such as mindful listening, team gratitude, and acts of kindness at work, and using positive communication strategies to create positive dental teams. We can also create HQC moments with our patients through talking to patients in authentic ways, such as sharing stories about our children or mutual points of interest. HQCs with patients help to foster trusting relationships, but equally as important, they make us feel energised. Furthermore, coaching, mentoring, and joining dental groups can increase our availability to these important HQCs.

- **Engagement at work:** We engage at work through the ability to use our strengths. These are positive parts of our personality that impact how we think, act, and feel. Examples include love of learning, leadership, teamwork, and compassion. Our signature strengths daily can help us boost our resilience and well-being. We can also use them to help overcome challenges. Engagement can also be encouraged through increasing moments of flow, for example, during dental procedures such as composite bonding, facial aesthetics, or orthodontics. To learn more about strengths and flow, see Chapter 10.

Resilience Seesaw for Dental Professionals

The resilience seesaw (Figure 3.3) illustrates how PERLE factors boost us towards positive mental health. Each PERLE pillar can be considered a protective factor in helping us thrive at work. The initial placement of the fulcrum is dependent on our genetic makeup but is influenced by the interplay between our risk, protective factors, and what is going on in our lives. When positive life experiences and protective factors outweigh negative experiences and risk factors, a dental professional's 'scale' tips towards positive mental health outcomes. Over time, the cumulative impact of positive life experiences and protective factors shifts the fulcrum position, making one more susceptible to achieving positive mental health, away from clinician burnout to engagement and flourishing.

SEE SAW OF RESILIENCE FOR DENTAL PROFESSIONALS

LOAD POSITIVE SIDE UP

PROTECTIVE FACTORS

RESILIENT MINDSET
OPTIMISTIC, COMPASSIONATE & GROWTH MINDSET

PURPOSE

LIFESTYLE
GOOD NUTRITION, SLEEP & EXERCISE

EMOTIONAL INTELLIGENCE
SELF AWARENESS
EMOTIONAL-REGULATION
POSITIVE EMOTIONS

ENVIRONMENT
HIGH QUALITY CONNECTIONS
USING STRENGTHS

POSITIVE MENTAL HEALTH OUTCOMES
E.G FLOURISHING

FULCRUM >>

<< FULCRUM >>

REDUCE RISK FACTORS

RISK FACTORS

LONELINESS

EMOTIONAL DYSREGULATION

DISENGAGEMENT AT WORK

LOW LEVELS OF PURPOSE

TOXIC WORK ENVIRONMENT

HIGH NEGATIVE EMOTIONS

POOR DIET, SLEEP & LOW EXERCISE

PESSIMISTIC, CRITICAL & FIXED MINDSETS

NEGATIVE MENTAL HEALTH OUTCOMES
E.G BURNOUT

MY MENTAL WELLNESS CHECK-IN

USE THESE REFLECTION PROMPTS AND SIMPLE STEPS, BASED ON PERLE, TO REGULARLY CHECK IN WITH YOUR OWN MENTAL WELLNESS AND YOUR TEAM

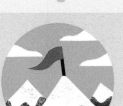

PURPOSE

DO I HAVE A SENSE OF MEANING IN MY LIFE?

- Which small and big moments with patients bring me meaning?
- How can I bring my values to my interactions with patients?
- How can I align my goals with my values?
- Which acts of kindness can I do at work today?
- What's the silver lining to my major challenge today?

EMOTIONAL INTELLIGENCE

HOW AM I FEELING TODAY?

- What's my internal weather?
- What is my current energy level today?
- Am I experiencing more positive or negative emotions? Am I stressed? Burnt out?
- Am I using helpful coping strategies to manage my stress?
- What brings me joy and how can I do more of it?
- What are 3 things, big or small, that went well for me this week?
- Which 3 things am I grateful for today?
- How can I increase mindfulness at work? E.g. mindful deep breaths whilst waiting curing composite!

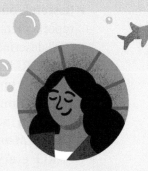

RESILIENT MINDSET

HOW'S MY THINKING TODAY?

- How are my thoughts making me feel?
- Are my thoughts helping or hindering me?
- How can I reframe challenges in dentistry with optimism?
- How can I remind myself that when 'failures' arise I can learn lessons and keep improving?
- Which growth mindset affirmations can I use during difficult or new treatment with patients?
- How can I respond with words and gestures of self-kindness in moments of stress today instead of self-criticism?

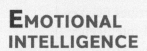

LIFESTYLE

HOW CAN I BOOST MY PHYSICAL WELL-BEING?

- Am I eating a balanced diet and drinking enough water?
- How am I able to get more movement in my day?
- Should I be prioritising my sleep tonight?

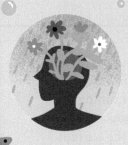
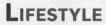

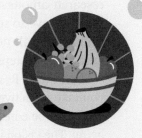

ENVIRONMENT

HOW CAN I FEEL CONNECTED WITH OTHERS AND MORE ENGAGED AT WORK?

- Where, when, and how can I increase my HQCs at work?
- How can I share gratitude with team members? Would I benefit from a mentor or coach?
- How can I use my strengths more with patients and at home?
- Can I schedule in protected time for referrals/admin in the patient diary?
- Can we designate a mental wellness lead for the team?

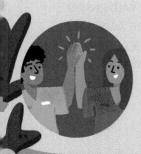

Summary

- Resilience is a journey where we use our inner psychological resources to overcome adversities.
- We can train our minds to become more resilient.
- Resilience training can provide many benefits to the dental team: greater ability to regulate emotions, handle crisis, enhance communication, improve relationships, and increase authenticity at work.
- Research on well-being and resilience training for medical professionals reports increases in well-being post-intervention.
- PTG describes a process of growth that can occur after adversities.
- The PERLE Resilience Model for Dental Professionals describes five key pillars of building resilience at work: **P**urpose, **E**motional intelligence, **R**esilient mindset, **L**ifestyle, and **E**nvironment at work. Increasing any pillar can increase levels of psychological resilience.
- The *My Mental Wellness Check-in* can help you and the dental team apply PERLE everyday and boost your resilience as a result

 The View From Here

Resilience is very much about how we learn to not just survive but to thrive when we experience setbacks. This is a dynamic process and one in which we grow through our challenges. The numerous benefits of resilience training for dental professionals points to clinician well-being being a necessary and important part of dental education early on. This is backed up by the current research amongst our medical and healthcare peers. And for this reason, I would love to see resilience in undergraduate curriculas, annual resilience training for all dental teams, and programmes helping dental professionals take positive steps forward.

The PERLE Resilience Model introduced in this chapter is designed to help you take proactive steps in becoming a more resilient dental professional. Each pillar can be considered as a protective factor in boosting positive mental well-being. The vision is to help you nurture your internal and external psychological reservoirs, so you can navigate any challenge or stressor in dentistry with greater ease. PERLE helps you invite more purpose; increase your self-awareness, your ability to regulate emotions, and your diet of positive emotions; grow optimistic, compassionate, and growth-thinking styles; lead a positive lifestyle; draw on HQCs; and use your strengths with patients and at home.

In subsequent chapters, we probe into the five pillars of the PERLE framework. Each chapter is full of practical tools for dental professionals interested in finding their inner strength, overcoming life's hurdles, and thriving in the process.

References

Aboalshamat, K., Hou, X.Y., and Strodl, E. (2015). Psychological well-being status among medical and dental students in Makkah, Saudi Arabia: a cross-sectional study. *Medical Teacher* 37 (Suppl 1): S75–S81.

Chapman, H., Chipchase, S., and Bretherton, R. (2017). The evaluation of a continuing professional development package for primary care dentists designed to reduce stress, build resilience and improve clinical decision-making. *British Dental Journal* 223: 261–271.

Clough, B.A., March, S., Chan, R.J. et al. (2017). Psychosocial interventions for managing occupational stress and burnout among medical doctors: a systematic review. *Systematic Reviews* 6 (1): 144.

Gònzalez, G. and Quezada, V.E. (2016). A brief cognitive-behavioral intervention for stress, anxiety and depressive symptoms in dental students. *Research in Psychotherapy: Psychopathology, Process and Outcome* 19 (1): 68–78.

Gorter, R. C. (2000). Burnout among dentists: Identification and prevention. Doctoral dissertation. Universiteit van Amsterdam.

Machado, L., de Oliveira, I.R., Peregrino, A., and Cantilino, A. (2019). Common mental disorders and subjective well-being: emotional training among medical students based on positive psychology. *PLoS One* 14 (2): e0211926.

Metz, C.J., Ballard, E., and Metz, M.J. (2020). The stress of success: an online module to help first-year dental students cope with the impostor phenomenon. *Journal of Dental Education* 84: 1016–1024.

Newton, J.T., Allen, C.D., Coates, J. et al. (2006). How to reduce the stress of general dental practice: the need for research into the effectiveness of multifaceted interventions. *British Dental Journal* 200: 437–440.

Peng, L., Li, M., Zuo, X. et al. (2014). Application of the Pennsylvania resilience training program on medical students. *Personality and Individual Differences* 61–62: 47–51.

Plessas, A., Paisi, M., Bryce, M. et al. (2021). Mental health and wellbeing in dentistry: a rapid evidence assessment. *General Dental Council.*.

Rosenzweig, S., Reibel, D.K., Greeson, J.M. et al (2003). Mindfulness-based stress reduction lowers psychological distress in medical students. Teaching and

Learning in Medicine, 15. https://www.tandfonline.com/doi/abs/10.1207/S15328015TLM1502_03

Smith, B.W., Dalen, J., Wiggins, K. et al. (2008). The brief resilience scale: assessing the ability to bounce back. *International Journal of Behavioral Medicine* 15 (3): 194–200.

Sood, A., Prasad, K., Schroeder, D., and Varkey, P. (2011). Stress management and resilience training among department of medicine faculty: a pilot randomized clinical trial. *Journal of General Internal Medicine* 26: 858–861.

4

Purpose: Honing the Practice of Making Meaning in Dentistry

CHAPTER OVERVIEW

- Benefits of purpose and meaning for dental professionals
- Understanding our core values
- Goal setting using values
- Acts of kindness
- Benefit finding.

> *Life is not primarily a quest for pleasure, as Freud believed, or a quest for power, as Alfred Alder taught, but a quest for meaning.*
>
> —Viktor Frankl

It is no wonder that the first pillar of the PERLE Resilience Model starts with 'P' for purpose. Having a sense of meaning brings immense richness to our everyday lives. As dental professionals, finding purpose in our work plays a crucial role in our engagement and satisfaction. Studies report lower levels of meaning relate to increased rates of burnout and compassion fatigue.

Having a sense of purpose in life can be defined as the degree to which people make sense of their lives and the world around them, perceiving their life to have inherent value and be worth living (Steger et al. 2021). We gain purpose from experiences, situations, big or small, and reflecting on the cosmic meaning of everything.

The search for meaning has been an important question pondered throughout history. Ancient Greek philosopher Socrates viewed the meaning of life as both personal and spiritual growth. For Plato, the meaning of life was knowledge. For Aristotle, the purpose of life was to achieve eudaimonia (happiness through the pursuit of meaning). The literature validates that high levels of meaning in individuals create happier people, healthier immune systems, more satisfying relationships, longer lives, and slower advancement of cognitive decline and Alzheimer's disease (Steger 2012; Roepke et al. 2014; Cohen et al. 2016; Alimujiang et al. 2019).

Resilience and Well-being for Dental Professionals, First Edition. Mahrukh Khwaja.
© 2023 John Wiley & Sons Ltd. Published 2023 by John Wiley & Sons Ltd.
Companion website: www.wiley.com/go/khwaja-resilience-dentistry

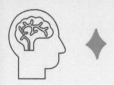

Think About It

Maslows Hierarchy of Needs

Did you know that having a strong sense of meaning is a human need? Maslow's hierarchy of needs is a five-tier model exploring our needs as humans. The bottom of the hierarchy incorporates our physiological needs (nutrition, sleep, clothing). The next level is our safety needs (security, protection, freedom from fear). Psychological needs form the next two levels of the pyramid: love and belonging (friendship, intimacy) and esteem needs (positive self-evaluation, prestige, feeling of accomplishment). Self-actualisation lies at the top of the pyramid. This need focuses on meaning, growth, transcendence, exploration, and play. The needs lower down the pyramid must be satisfied before individuals can proceed to the needs higher up. In the West, our basic needs of food, shelter, and security are often met, as well as our psychological needs of belonging and feeling of accomplishment. This leaves us in a position to really consider the highest human need of creating a life that also deeply excites us, nourishes our curiosity, is rich and meaningful, and in which we emotionally grow.

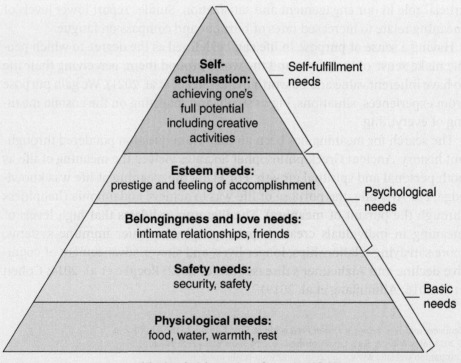

Maslow's hierarchy of needs (1943).

There are many routes to finding purpose in dentistry. In this chapter, we explore three strategies: using your core values as a dental professional, practising acts of kindness at work, and finding meaning in stressful times.

Using Our Core Values at Work

Understanding our core values as dental professionals can help us navigate a long, purposeful dental career. Our values can also help us manage difficult situations at work, such as a challenging, aggressive patient. Research on values-based health-care points to benefits of our patients feeling cared for, respected, and having trust in us. Working with our patients and doing things that are incongruent with our core values can contribute to negative feelings towards work. Burnout and compassion fatigue seem also to be impacted by value incongruence. A large Canadian study of more than 8000 participants reported that workload and value incongruence predicted burnout amongst physicians (Leiter et al. 2009). The interplay between values and workload in women had greater consequences than men in their study, with greater levels of burnout. Clarifying our core values allows us to better define our roles and expectations in the dental field. We can engage more fully and shape how we show up in the spaces we work in.

A life full of rarely lived values can feel stifling. When we live our values and express our strengths, work and our personal life become both joyful and meaningful.

But what are values? And how do they differ from goals? Our values are our heart's deepest desires in how we want to treat ourselves and others. They are what we stand for in life and give us meaning and purpose. We can think of them as our inner compass to choose effective actions. Translating our values to effective action – action that is aligned with who we are and what matters the most – requires us to really understand what we stand for. Without this, when we are disconnected from our values, we can act in ways that are incongruent from the ways we want to be in life. Living life guided by our values, on the other hand, allows us to feel more engaged and experience life as rich and meaningful.

We spend a lot of our time as a society thinking about our goals. Values are not the same as goals: values are how we want to behave and goals are things we want to achieve. Examples of values we use with our patients at work include patient centeredness, integrity, respect, compassion, kindness, professionalism, teamwork, support, and service. Values provide a direction we want to keep moving in. When we align our values with our goals, our motivation becomes supercharged, known as 'intrinsic motivation'. This is a, psychologically speaking, good type of motivation that will help us stick to our habits in the longer term; for example, if connecting with nature is a value, you'll prioritise taking a nature walk, or if self-care is important, you're more likely to exercise and prioritise good nutrition.

Think About It

Identifying Your Values

Have a look at the table of values from Acceptance and Commitment Therapy. Which values at work resonate with you the most? Which values reflect you in your personal life? Pick your top five values and reflect on why these specific values matter.

Accountability	Diversity	Humility	Security
Accuracy	Dynamism	Independence	Self-actualization
Achievement	Economy	Ingenuity	Self-control
Adventurousness	Effectiveness	Inner harmony	Selflessness
Altruism	Efficiency	Inquisitiveness	Sell-reliance
Ambition	Elegance	Insightfulness	Sensitivity
Assertiveness	Empathy	Intelligence	Serenity
Balance	Enjoyment	Intellectual status	Service
Belonging	Enthusiasm	Intuition	Shrewdness
Boldness	Equality	Joy	Simplicity
Calmness	Excellence	Justice	Soundness
Carefulness	Excitement	Leadership	Speed
Challenge	Expertise	Legacy	Spontaneity
Cheerfulness	Exploration	Love	Stability
Commitment	Expressiveness	Loyalty	Strategic
Community	Fairness	Making a difference	Strength
Compassion	Faith	Mastery	Structure
Competitiveness	Fidelity	Merit	Success
Consistency	Fitness	Obedience	Support
Contentment	Fluency	Openness	Teamwork
Contribution	Focus	Order	Temperance
Control	Freedom	Originality	Thankfulness
Cooperation	Fun	Patriotism	Thoroughness
Correctness	Generosity	Perfection	Thoughtfulness
Courtesy	Goodness	Piety	Timeliness
Creativity	Grace	Positivity	Tolerance
Curiosity	Growth	Practicality	Traditionalism
Decisiveness	Happiness	Preparedness	Trustworthiness
Dependability	Hard Work	Professionalism	Truth-seeking
Determination	Health	Prudence	Understanding
Devoutness	Helping Society	Quality-orientation	Uniqueness
Diligence	Holiness	Reliability	Usefulness
Discipline	Honesty	Resourcefulness	Vision
Discretion	Honor	Restraint	Vitality

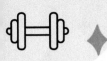

Setting Values-based Goals

1. Write down your top five values below that resonate with you the most at work and in your personal life.

2. Now consider how your top five goals relate to each life quadrant below, and write these in the corresponding quadrant. How do your goals align with your values?

Dental career

Relationships

Health

Leisure

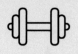

Setting Values-based Goals

3. List short-, medium-, and long-term goals, keeping your top values in mind. Which small steps can you take to reach these goals? Include a schedule for when you will do it. Enlist support from friends and family. This table can be your action plan in achieving your goals, based on what matters to you the most.

Short-term goals	Medium-term goals	Long-term goals

Practising Acts of Kindness

We can also invite purpose through doing small and big acts of kindness; that is, aligning ourselves to a cause bigger than ourselves, from charities to helping our colleagues. Positive psychology research shows that doing small acts of kindness, from paying someone a compliment at work or allowing someone to go ahead of you in a queue, is good for us as well as for the recipients. In fact, some studies have reported that performing just one random act of kindness a day can reduce stress and anxiety, and your body is flooded with the hormones we discussed earlier, which make you feel calmer, healthier, and happier. Random acts of kindness can also promote a phenomenon known as the 'happiness contagion', where one good deed causes others to continue the chain of good deeds! It doesn't take much, but it does make a difference.

Benefits of Random Acts of Kindness

- **Reduce isolation**: Acts of kindness encourage us to connect with the community and engage with others.
- **Reduce pain**: Kindness produces endorphins – the brain's natural pain killer.
- **Reduce blood pressure:** Kindness generates emotional warmth, which causes the release of oxytocin. This helps to lower blood pressure and improve overall cardiovascular health.
- **Reduce anxiety**: Stimulation of serotonin helps lift our mood
- **Reduce stress.**

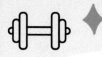

Culture Of Kindness At Work

The research on kind work cultures is growing, with studies showing that these workspaces are more productive and profitable than negative work cultures. In a long perspective study of 11 years, positive cultures had stock growth 10 times greater than organisations with negative work cultures (Kotter 2008). Try this one-month challenge to introduce more random acts of kindness and enjoyment at work.

- Play gratitude 'ping-pong', passing a ball back and fro listing things you are grateful for.
- Offer a helping hand to a colleague.
- Listen to learn, not to respond.
- Put your phone away when you're talking to a colleague.
- Be thoughtful in how you respond to others, and be mindful of their perspective.
- Invite someone at work you would like a stronger connection with to lunch.
- Befriend a new work colleague.
- Bake a cake and take it into work to show your gratitude for the team.
- Keep common areas clean and tidy.
- Make a cup of tea for a colleague.
- If someone had a good idea in a meeting, tell the person so.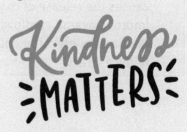
- Leave a note of appreciation.
- Choose to smile more.
- Become a mentor.
- Write positive sticky notes for a colleague.
- Remembering birthdays and work-iversaries.
- Forgive mistakes and look for ways to help colleagues improve.
- Offer to do someone's least favourite task.
- Gift a book that has inspired you.
- Send an encouraging message to a colleague.
- Leave a positive recommendation on LinkedIn.
- Organise a leaving collection or a special occasion collection.
- Bring treats to a team meeting.
- Avoid negative chatter about colleagues.
- Spread good news and ask your colleagues about what is going well in their lives.

If you are interested in helping your community, you may want to explore local charity organisations. One example includes the Random Acts of Kindness Foundation. This has plenty of kindness ideas as well as the opportunity to become a Random Acts of Kindness Activist, a kindness ambassador organising community projects and monthly kindness challenges.

Benefit Finding

During challenges at work, having a sense of purpose is a key player in regulating our emotions and helping us to employ effective coping strategies. In terms of the mechanism in which purpose works, the research points to meaning having both buffering and building effects when it comes to our mental well-being. Research even during the Covid-19 pandemic spotlighted that meaning in life during the pandemic buffers against Covid-19 specific stress (Trzebiński et al. 2020) as well as depression and anxiety (Chao et al. 2020).

If we can find benefits in the challenges we face in dentistry, we are much more likely to weather negative life circumstances and even grow through them. A particularly useful exercise that can strengthen our levels of purpose is a journaling activity, known as benefit finding.

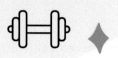

Benefit Finding

1. Reflect on a recent challenge or adversity you have experienced over the last year. How did you view the world, and what were your beliefs about yourself and your identity preadversity?

2. Consider how you have made sense of the change and the journey to discover new avenues to meaning. What big and small moments in your day enhance your sense of meaning in life?

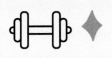
3. How you have grown through this time?

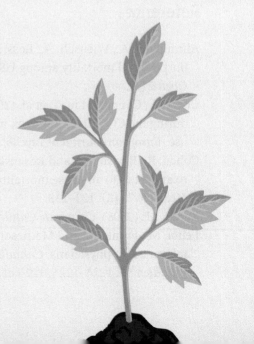

Summary

- There are many benefits to meaning: physical health, mental health, and reduced risk of depression and antisocial behaviour.
- Meaning can be increased through using values at work, aligning our goals with these values, small or big acts of kindness, and the benefit-finding exercise.
- We can use values tables, such as from Acceptance and Commitment Therapy, or journaling to reflect on what our values are.

 The View From Here

By delving into the 'P' of the PERLE Resilience Model, we begin to appreciate how having a sense of purpose is the secret sauce in helping us feel good, more engaged, and optimistic and in living a life that is rich and meaningful. Meaning making requires us to make this pillar a real priority: to reflect on our core values and bring them to work with our patients, to create goals that align with what matters the most to us, to practise acts of kindness, big and small, and to seek the silver linings in our daily challenges in dentistry. As Viktor Frankl so beautifully put it: 'The meaning of life is to give life meaning'.

References

Alimujiang, A., Wiensch, A., Boss, J. et al. (2019). Association between life purpose and mortality among US adults older than 50 years. *JAMA Network Open* 2 (5).

Chao, M., Chen, X., Liu, T. et al. (2020). Psychological distress and state boredom during the COVID-19 outbreak in China: the role of meaning in life and media use. *European Journal of Psychotraumatology* 11 (1): 1769379.

Cohen, R., Bavishi, C., and Rosanski, A. (2016). Purpose in life and its relationship to all-cause mortality and cardiovascular events. *Psychosomatic Medicine* 78 (2): 122–133.

Kotter, J.P. (2008). *Corporate Culture and Performance*. Simon and Schuster.

Leiter, M., Frank, E., and Matheson, T. (2009). Demands, values, and burnout relevance for physicians. *Canadian Family Physician Médecin de famille canadien* 55: 1224–1225, 1225.e1.

Roepke, A.M., Jayawickreme, E., and Riffle, O.M. (2014). Meaning and health: a systematic review. *Applied Research in Quality of Life* 9 (4): 1055–1079.

Steger, M.F. (2012). Making meaning in life. *Psychological Inquiry* 23 (4): 381–385.

Steger, M.F., O'Donnell, M.B., and Morse, J.L. (2021). Helping students find their way to meaning: meaning and purpose in education. In: *The Palgrave Handbook of Positive Education*, 551–579. Cham, Switzerland: Palgrave Macmillan.

Trzebiński, J., Cabański, M., and Czarnecka, J.Z. (2020). Reaction to the COVID-19 pandemic: the influence of meaning in life, life satisfaction, and assumptions on world orderliness and positivity. *Journal of Loss and Trauma* 25: 544–577.

5

Developing Emotional Intelligence

CHAPTER OVERVIEW

- Emotional intelligence benefits for dental professionals
- What are emotions?
- Measure your level of emotions
- Science of positive emotions
- Power of positivity ratio
- Broaden-and-Build Theory
- Personality and emotions
- Mind tools to help regulate emotions.

By teaching people to tune into their emotions with intelligence and expand their circles of caring, we can transform organizations from the inside out and make a positive difference in our world.

—Daniel Goleman, psychologist, author, and journalist

Emotional intelligence (EI), also known as emotional quotient or EQ, is the ability to monitor our own and others' feelings and emotions, to discriminate among them, and to use this information to guide our own thinking and actions (Salovey and Mayer 1990). High EI allows us to understand what we and others are feeling, regulate our emotions in positive ways to relieve stress, communicate effectively, empathise with others, and defuse conflict.

The first 'E' of the PERLE model spotlights emotional intelligence and its crucial role in building resilience. This is split into three interplaying parts: self-awareness, emotional regulation, and positive emotions. Due to the sheer vastness of this pillar and topic, we explore EI over three chapters.

Tuning to our emotions with intelligence is critical for dental professionals. Our emotions drive our every behaviour. And as the old adage goes in dentistry, patients do not remember what we say but rather how we make them feel. In this chapter, we will explore the transformative benefits of developing EI for dental professionals and how to do so.

Resilience and Well-being for Dental Professionals, First Edition. Mahrukh Khwaja.
© 2023 John Wiley & Sons Ltd. Published 2023 by John Wiley & Sons Ltd.
Companion website: www.wiley.com/go/khwaja-resilience-dentistry

EI Benefits in Dentistry

Benefits of High Emotional Intelligence for Dental Professionals
- Increased empathy
- Better quality of patient care
- Greater work engagement
- Greater career satisfaction
- Improved leadership, teamwork, and communication.

Developing high EI has numerous advantages for dental professionals. Self-awareness – that is, knowing how we are feeling – and emotion regulation, the ability to downregulate from stress to calm, helps us build greater resilience and psychological well-being. The ability to manage our emotional life without being hijacked by it is a tremendous learnable skill. With it, we are better equipped to respond well under the pressures of dentistry. High EI leads ultimately to us developing increased empathy with our patients, resulting in better quality of patient care. Recognising emotions in our patients and attempting to understand how they are influencing behaviours is one of the building blocks of empathy. Furthermore, greater connection to patients enhances our levels of engagement at work and hence career satisfaction.

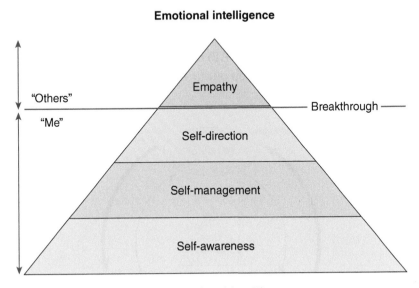

Facets of Emotional Intelligence

Additionally, high EI is essential for effective communication, leadership, and teamwork. Ensuring patients understand the information we are conveying to them is essential for obtaining valid informed consent and for building strong patient relationships that may prevent or reduce the risk of complaints. The ability to recognise by facial expression when a patient is anxious or confused allows a dental professional to pause the consultation and explore any questions or concerns before continuing.

Guiding Principles of Developing Emotional Intelligence
- **Self-awareness:** Make it a habit to check in with your emotions.
- **Curious attitude:** Be curious, patient, and non-judgmental with your emotions.
- **Increase your emotional literacy:** Use emotion wheels to increase range of vocabulary describing emotions.
- **Authenticity:** Talk about and show your real emotions.
- **Acceptance:** No emotion is bad, it just is. Learn to accept having different emotions.

What are Emotions?

Emotions are pieces of information that tell us something about how we are experiencing our world. Emotions are often feared and avoided, as they can be painful; however, they are designed to help us survive, relate to other people, communicate how we feel, and respond to our world. Emotions give us feedback on our environment, that is, whether it is dangerous or friendly. They tell us what we need so that we take action to meet our needs. They also are influenced by our thoughts or perceptions and can trigger physical responses and behaviours. All emotions are forms of energy that drive our behaviours. This is explained through the cognitive-behavioural therapy (CBT) model (see Figure 5.1) that conveys the interconnected relationship between our feelings, thoughts, and actions.

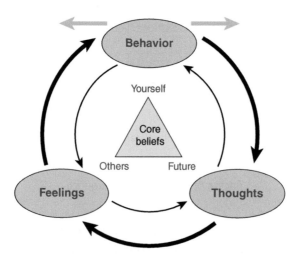

Figure 5.1 The CBT model. Source: Adapted from Beck 1964 and Ellis 1957.

Our emotional reaction was learnt from our childhood experiences. If we were predominantly fearful as a child, we may overprotect ourself as an adult, and this may present as anxiety. Emotions are also modified by the genetic makeup of a person (temperament) and the socialisation process.

Taking Off the Mask

With our patient-focused role in dentistry, we need to keep some of our emotions and feelings under the surface and lean into a calm, compassionate, empathetic, and confident state. Although this is of course necessary, it is important, outside our time with patients, to experience our emotions with acceptance and non-judgment and release them. Keeping our feelings bottled up can cause us to blow up or develop stress-related illnesses. Pushing down feelings only means they will resurface at a later date.

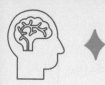

Think About It

Label Your Emotions

What emotions have you experienced in the past 24 hours at work? What emotions do you experience most often and how do you express them? What triggers your emotional reactions? Patients, places, times, or words?

Emotion	Percentage of the day	What was the trigger?
Anger		
Disgust		
Fear		
Joy		
Sadness		
Surprise		

Think About It

Increase Your Emotional Literacy

Use the emotional wheel below to reflect on your different emotions and increase your vocabulary around how you felt today.

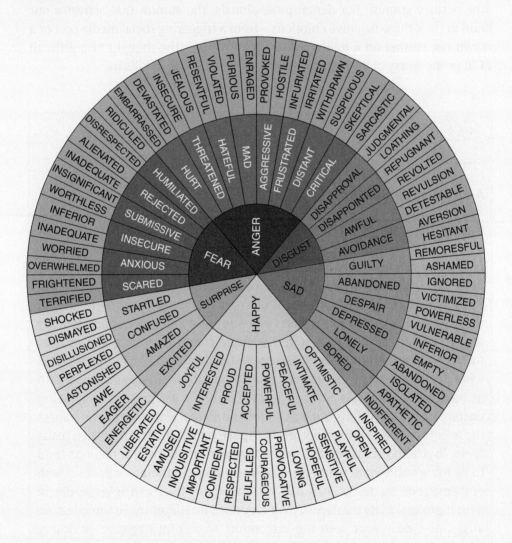

Paul Ekman (2003) identified six basic human emotions found across age, gender, and culture, with some emotions arousing you and others calming you down. These include anger, disgust, fear, joy, sadness, and surprise. Our feelings arise from our basic emotions. There are more unpleasant emotions than pleasant. As mentioned in Chapters 1 and 2 ('the negativity bias'), from an evolutionary standpoint, that makes sense. The benefits of negative emotions elicited by real or potential danger meant that our thought-action repertoire was narrowed, and therefore fear would elicit the action of running away and anger lead to us defending ourselves in battle. Humans also have a tendency towards negative over positive stimuli. For dental professionals, the stimuli that activates our brain to elicit these negative emotions – from a triggering social media post or a crown not seating on a tooth, a difficult extraction, the thought of a difficult RCT, or the worry of an impending exam – is not going to kills us.

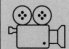

Learning From Movies

A Case Study: Inside Out

Disney Pixar's movie *Inside Out* beautifully brings Ekman's model of basic emotions to life and the concept of EI. It tells the story of 11-year-old Riley navigating a move across the country and how the basic emotions, as described by Ekman, balance the control of her mind, from a mission control headquarters. Each day consists of discreet moments coloured by one of these emotions. The real fun starts when Joy and Sadness get accidentally ejected out of headquarters, and the movie charts their cathartic journey through other mental areas of her brain. The pivotal point in the movie is when Joy realises that Sadness is just as important for Riley's mental health as happiness. *Inside Out* makes the case of the importance of embracing uncomfortable emotions, such as sadness and fear – to accept and expect these emotions and allow yourself the space to feel them rather than resist them. Psychologists have discovered that our emotions and feelings tend to be more unpleasant when we suppress them, and therefore dealing with our emotions by acceptance and making room for them is essential in dental professionals mastering their emotions intelligently. So the question arises, how do we sit with the discomfort of painful negative emotions, such as fear, with courage and acceptance? In the next sections, we will explore the mind tools to do so.

The Broadening Effect of Positive Emotions

What do positive emotions do to our thinking? Barbara Fredrickson, leading researcher in positive emotions, has been studying this area with avid interest. Her Broaden and Build Theory (Fredrickson 2001), backed up with research, describes the transformative effects of positive emotions on our success and well-being. The experience of positive emotions, from joy to serenity, gratitude, awe, inspiration, and amusement, opens our minds and broadens our ability to think 'outside the box' (Figure 5.2). Our outlook on our environment changes. The world appears larger. We see more possibilities relative to negative or neutral states. This is the opposite case for stress, in which our thinking considerably narrows.

The broadening effect of positive emotions in turn helps us to build personal resources when we need them: intellectual (problem solving, open to learning), physical (cardiovascular health, coordination), social (maintain relationships and create new ones), and psychological (resilience, optimism, sense of identity and goal orientation) (see Figure 5.2). This in turns helps us transform our lives. Interestingly, the impact of positive emotions extends beyond us just feeling better, as they can impact our physical health. Positive emotions can 'undo cardiovascular after effects of negativity' (Fredrickson 2009). Positive emotions can help our bodies return to normal physiological functioning significantly faster than other emotions (Fredrickson and Levenson 1998).

Evidence-Based Benefits of Positive Emotions
Broaden our thinking
Build psychological resources
Build intellectual resources
Build physical resources
Build social resources
Spiral of further positive emotions
More creativity
Better academic performance
Physicians make better medical decisions (Isen et al. 1991)
Look past racial difference and see towards oneness.

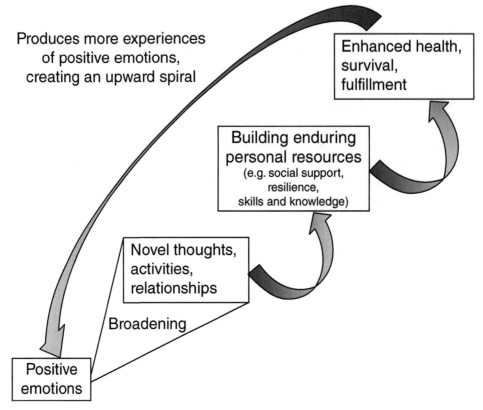

Figure 5.2 The Broaden-and-Build Theory (Fredrickson 2004).

Think About It

Positive Emotions

What positive emotions have you experienced in the last 24 hours? What were the triggers? What can you do to cultivate these feelings more?

Emotion	Percentage of the day	What was the trigger?
Joy		
Gratitude		
Serenity		
Interest		
Surprise		
Hope		
Pride		
Amusement		
Inspiration		
Awe		
Love		

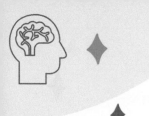

Think About It

Our Emotional Tank

A useful metaphor for thinking about positive emotions is comparing it to the tank of fuel in one's car. We need to replenish our levels of positive emotions, the fuel that keeps us going and helps us to thrive and flourish. Fredrickson's research identified that the number of positive emotions to negative ratio for thriving is 3:1. Interestingly, the data show that most people have a ratio more towards 2:1.

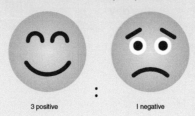

3 positive   I negative

Personality and Emotion

Which personality traits bring us all together? Which traits separate us as individuals? Personality psychology can give us insight into this and acknowledges the individual differences in how we think, feel, and act. The most widely used personality test comes from research by Costa and McRae (1992). They identified five main personality traits across cultures, known as the Big Five. Table 5.1 summarises these traits. How do you think you would score on each trait?

Table 5.1   Big Five trait summaries.

Extraversion	**High scorers:** Tend to respond positively to stimuli in the outside world. Feel energised after speaking to a lot of people.
	Low scorers: Focus inwards, drained after speaking to lots of people, tend to be quieter, shy, and prefer to be alone.
Agreeableness	**High scorers:** Tend to likeable, patient with others, let go of angry feelings quicker, compassionate, and sympathetic to others' needs.
	Low scorers: Untrusting, critical, and suspicious.
Conscientiousness	**High scorers:** Pay attention to detail, plan every detail. Tend to have high levels of grit and are diligent, efficient, and reliable.
	Low scorers: Inattentive, idle, sometimes unreliable.
Neuroticism	**High scorers:** High levels of anxiety, insecurity, tend to experience higher highs and lower lows.
	Low scorers: Tranquil, steady, and composed.
Openness to experience	**High scorers:** Curious about the world around them and are open to trying new things. Tend to like being creative and exploring alternative ideas.
	Low scorers: Don't like to break out of their comfort zone. Tend to be conformist and uncreative.

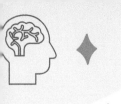

Think About It

The Big Five

There is a strong correlation between positive emotions and well-being with extroversion (Costa and McRae 1980; Shiota et al. 2006), whereas neuroticism is associated with depression and lower levels of well-being. Conscientiousness has been shown to be associated with joy, contentment, and pride. When we are designing our own well-being interventions – that is, trying out different well-being activities for a period of time – it is worth tailor-making them to our personality type for maximum potential. Try the free Big Five assessment to learn more about your own personality traits at https://bigfive-test.com/.

EI and Well-being

EI can be thought of as a behaviour and a personality trait. It is impacted by several factors-our personality, attachment style we formed as children, and content and the context of a situation. Higher EI correlates to higher subjective well-being. Our EI does change and adapt over time, perhaps being influenced by the positivity bias as we age. The data suggest that our happiness levels increase as EI increases, such as positively reframing our emotional experiences. High EI is positively related with subjective well-being; mediated by emotional regulation strategies, such as emotional savouring (reliving positive emotions).

The Roadmap to EI

The most supported theory on emotional intelligence comes from the pioneering work of Mayer and Salovey (2007) and their theory on EI. This model considers developing EI as a set of competencies or mental skills that consist of four stages, as shown in Figure 5.3. The stages are summarised below.

Four stages of EI	Questions to ask yourself to develop mental skills
Perceiving: Ability to recognise emotions in yourself and others. Individuals are better equipped for social circumstances.	How do you feel? How do others feel?
Using emotions: Use emotions to facilitate mood.	How does your mood influence your thinking? How is it affecting your decision-making?
Understanding emotions.	Why are you feeling this? What do these emotions mean? What has triggered this for you?
Managing emotions: Manage and self-regulate emotions.	Identify when it's inappropriate to express certain emotions until the appropriate time

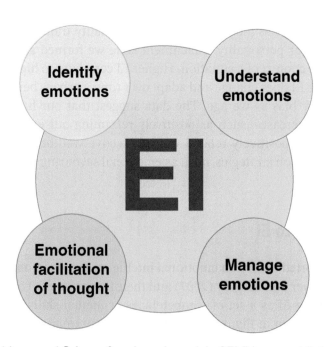

Figure 5.3 Mayer and Salovey four-branch model of EI (Mayer and Salovey 2007).

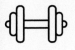

The Mind Gym: Your Guide to Regulating Emotions

In this section, learn practical ways of applying the theory to your own life:

- Select the right mind gym tools for you
- Explore the mind gym menu
- Try out the Mind-Flossing Exercises.

We will explore how to regulate difficult emotions and build greater resilience and well-being, using emotional coping tools. Table 5.2 summarises different tools we can select. Some strategies are generally considered to be helpful, such as expressing our feelings, mindfulness, self-compassion, physical exercise, or problem solving, and others mainly unhelpful, for example, alcohol, avoidance, or rumination.

Emotional regulation is the effort to influence which emotions we feel, express, and play out. The key with learning the mind tools to regulate emotions is to understand the range of well-being strategies and experiment with the ones that can help you. This involves reading and understanding the demands of situation and selecting the appropriate emotional regulation skills. Social and cultural contexts also matter. We have to be flexible in the way we use these strategies. Which helpful and unhelpful strategies from Table 5.2 do you already use?

Table 5.2 Tools for regulating emotions.

Strategy	Helpful?	What is it?	How?	Evidence
Mindfulness	≫	Paying attention to thoughts and feelings, non-judgmentally.	1) Get comfortable. 2) Set a time limit. 3) Close your eyes. 4) Notice your body. 5) Feel your breath. 6) Notice mind has wandered. 7) Gently nudge attention back to breath kindly, as you would a young child.	Galante et al. (2018) – 616 Cambridge University students during exam time. Half had eight-week mindfulness course and the others had normal university support. The mindfulness group had reduced stress during exam period.
Acceptance	≫	Nonjudgmental acceptance and tolerance of emotions and negative thoughts. Acceptance predicts lower negative emotions and overlaps with mindfulness.	• Let your emotions be. • Let yourself have emotions without trying to change them. • There is nothing wrong with having certain emotions. • Let them run their course. For example, 'hello sadness...there you are...you come and go'. Or 'it's alright to be anxious...just let it be...it will die down eventually'. • Try not to judge your thoughts and emotions. • My thoughts and emotions don't mean I am good or bad – they just are what they are. They are like clouds passing through my mind. They do not reflect the truth about the world and about me.	Ford et al. (2017) studied 1000 participants. Individuals who accepted rather than judged their mental experiences and emotions had higher well-being and lower depression and anxiety.

Self-compassion 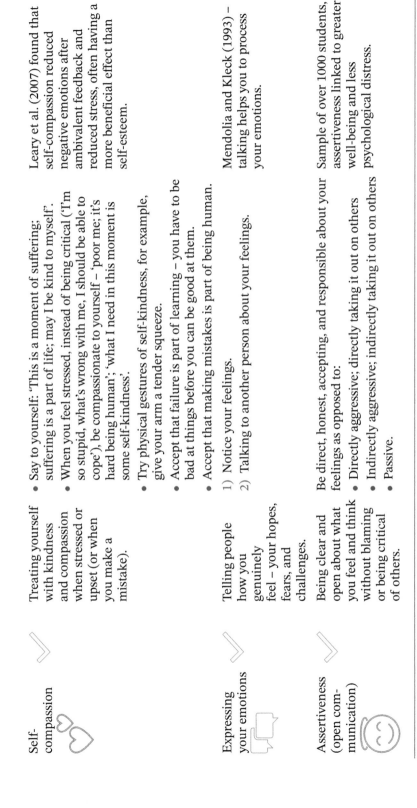	Treating yourself with kindness and compassion when stressed or upset (or when you make a mistake).	• Say to yourself: 'This is a moment of suffering; suffering is a part of life; may I be kind to myself'. • When you feel stressed, instead of being critical ('I'm so stupid, what's wrong with me, I should be able to cope'), be compassionate to yourself – 'poor me; it's hard being human'; 'what I need in this moment is some self-kindness'. • Try physical gestures of self-kindness, for example, give your arm a tender squeeze. • Accept that failure is part of learning – you have to be bad at things before you can be good at them. • Accept that making mistakes is part of being human.	Leary et al. (2007) found that self-compassion reduced negative emotions after ambivalent feedback and reduced stress, often having a more beneficial effect than self-esteem.
Expressing your emotions	Telling people how you genuinely feel – your hopes, fears, and challenges.	1) Notice your feelings. 2) Talking to another person about your feelings.	Mendolia and Kleck (1993) – talking helps you to process your emotions.
Assertiveness (open communication)	Being clear and open about what you feel and think without blaming or being critical of others.	Be direct, honest, accepting, and responsible about your feelings as opposed to: • Directly aggressive; directly taking it out on others • Indirectly aggressive; indirectly taking it out on others • Passive.	Sample of over 1000 students, assertiveness linked to greater well-being and less psychological distress.

(Continued)

Table 5.2 (Continued)

Strategy	Helpful?	What is it?	How?	Evidence
Cognitive reappraisal	⟩	Generating more helpful interpretations of a situation, for example, thinking of a failure as an opportunity to learn. This is most beneficial where we have limited control or no control, for example, grief/loss.	• Look at the evidence for and against the thought. • Ask yourself what you would say to a friend who thought this. • Ask yourself if the belief is helpful or unhelpful. • Zoom out of the situation; what will you think about this thought in a year's time? Does having this thought mean it's true?	Gross (1998) – reappraisal decreased emotional arousal in participants.
Exposure (feel the fear and do it anyway)	⟩	Deliberately exposing yourself to feared situation.	1) Find something that causes you anxiety. 2) Experiment with doing this and thinking; 'I'll feel the fear and do it anyway'. If this is difficult to do in one go, try building up to it in smaller steps.	Sloan and Telch (2002).
Physical exercise	⟩	Physical exertion that raises your heart rate.	• Even short periods of time exercising can boost your mood. • For more long-term mood benefits from exercise: aerobic and/or strength-building exercise for about 30 minutes three times a* week.	Stathopoulou et al. (2006) – exercise had a beneficial effect on mental health, including reducing depression and anxiety.

Problem solving	The process of finding solutions to difficult or complex issues.	Use when you are in a stressful situation that is within your control. 1) Brainstorm all possible solutions and write them down. Be creative, and nothing is off the table. 2) Evaluate the pros and cons of each option. Give each option a score out of 10. 3) Choose an option and do it. 4) See what happens – if your chosen option does not work, go back to steps 2 and 3 and choose a different option.	Cuijpers et al. (2007) – problem solving interventions helped to decrease depression.
Pleasure and mastery	A technique to help with low mood, pleasure and mastery is a way of planning your day to make sure you include things you find pleasurable and things you find give you a sense of achievement.	1) Write a list of things that give you pleasure. 2) Write a list of things that give you a sense of achievement (mastery). This second list can just be things you have to do but find hard— for example, chores. 3) Plan your day with a mixture of pleasure and mastery. For example, if you have to write an essay (mastery), intersperse, say, one hour of essay writing with one hour of doing something pleasurable, across the day, so you have, for example, three sessions of pleasure and three sessions of mastery.	Jacobson et al. (1996) – activating pleasure and mastery significantly lowered depression.

Table 5.2 (Continued)

Strategy	Helpful?	What is it?	How?	Evidence
Suppression	Mainly unhelpful	Hiding emotional states around others and yourself by pushing away the thoughts and emotions. It may be a short-term helpful strategy but not helpful long term. The opposite of suppression is authenticity – we are comfortable expressing our emotional states.	Use instead. . . • Mindfulness • Reappraisal • Acceptance • Self-compassion • Talking about your emotions.	Najmi et al. (2014) – OCD sufferers who were asked to suppress their negative OCD thought, actually thought about it more and were more distressed by it than OCD sufferers who were asked to accept their negative thought
Avoidance	Mainly unhelpful	Avoiding situations that lead to negative feelings. This can be a positive short-term strategy where we lack control but poor long-term strategy, as it does not address the causal experience.	Try. . . • Exposure – do something that you find scary and want to avoid. The more you do it, the less scary it will become. You can combine exposure with. . . • Acceptance – 'it's OK to feel anxious' • Self-compassion – 'good for me – I'm finding this difficult and that's tough – but aren't I doing well to face it when it's so hard?'	Aldao et al. (2010) – avoidance was associated with increases in depression and anxiety.

Rumination 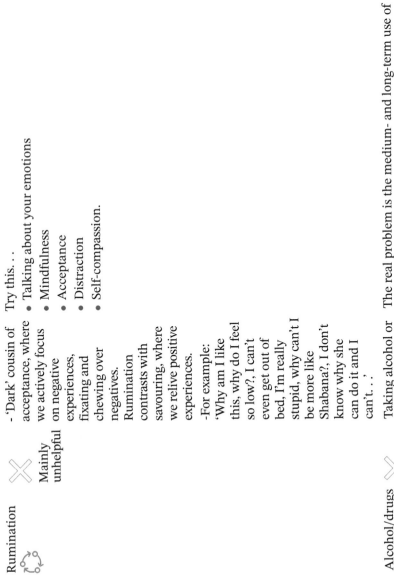	Mainly unhelpful	-'Dark' cousin of acceptance, where we actively focus on negative experiences, fixating and chewing over negatives. Rumination contrasts with savouring, where we relive positive experiences. -For example: 'Why am I like this, why do I feel so low?, I can't even get out of bed, I'm really stupid, why can't I be more like Shabana?, I don't know why she can do it and I can't. . .'	Try this. . . • Talking about your emotions • Mindfulness • Acceptance • Distraction • Self-compassion.	Nolen-Hoeksema and Morrow (1993) – depressed people who were asked to ruminate became more distressed, but those who were asked to use distraction (thinking about geographical locations) became less depressed. Broderick (2005) replicated Nolen-Hoeksema and Morrow's (1993) research but with an added mindfulness meditation condition of self-acceptance and awareness of the breath. This worked even better at reducing negative mood.
Alcohol/drugs	Mainly unhelpful	Taking alcohol or other substances to cope with emotions.	The real problem is the medium- and long-term use of drugs for emotion regulation.	Sher and Grekin (2007) – review of the negative effects of alcohol in emotion regulation.

(Continued)

Table 5.2 (Continued)

Strategy	Helpful?	What is it?	How?	Evidence
Self-criticism	✗	Attacking yourself when stressed or having a problem – for example, blaming yourself, or labelling yourself negatively.	For example, telling yourself 'I'm so lazy, I can't do anything', or 'I'm such an idiot – I really messed that up' normally has demotivating effects – so it doesn't help you to 'work harder'. And it makes you feel worse. Try... • Self-compassion • Mindfulness.	Gilbert and Procter (2006) – overview of the role of self-criticism in psychological difficulties.

The *Mind Gym* fitness menu below is a guide for helpful techniques to manage difficult emotions. Select options from the *Mind Gym* when you want help in coping with difficult emotions.

MIND GYM

Your Quick Guide for Managing Emotions

Select a mind work out to help support you with these common negative emotion:

Mind Workouts:

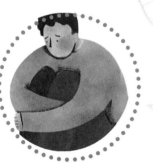

FEELING ANXIOUS

- Self-compassion
- Cognitive re-appraisal
- Exposure
- Acceptance
- Mindfulness
- Talking

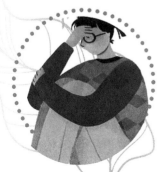

FEELING LOW

- Physical exercise
- Pleasure & mastery
- Self-compassion
- Talking

Source: Lasse Kristensen / Adobe Stock.

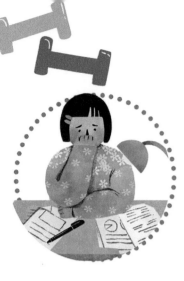

PROCASTINATION

- Self-compassion
- Mindfulness
- Acceptance
- Cognitive re-appraisal

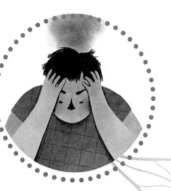

OVERWHELM

- Self-compassion
- Mindfulness
- Acceptance
- Cognitive re-appraisal
- Talking

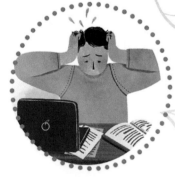

FEELING STRESSED

- Problem solving
- Pyhsical exercise
- Acceptance
- Mindfulness

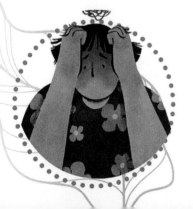

FEELING SOCIALLY ANXIOUS

- Assertiveness
- Exposure
- Self-compassion

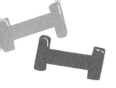

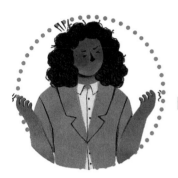

FEELING ANGRY

- Problem solving
- Pyhsical exercise
- Acceptance
- Mindfulness

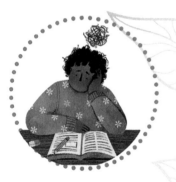

FEELING LIKE YOU'RE NOT GOOD ENOUGH

- Self-compassion
- Mindfulness
- Cognitive re-appraisal

Source: Lasse Kristensen / Adobe Stock.

Lifting the Mask of Self-Doubt: Managing Imposter Syndrome

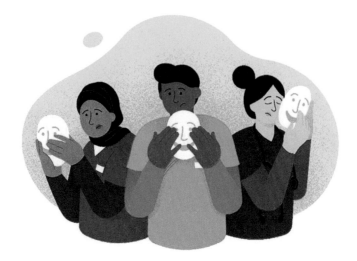

When did you last hear that voice at the back of your mind tell you are not good enough? That you have managed to fool everyone around you? Imposter syndrome is a set of negative thoughts and beliefs around your capabilities. This can really undermine your resilience and impact career progression. Imposter syndrome can feel like wearing a mask to prevent others finding out your 'true' competencies. For some colleagues, the more they accomplish, the more they feel like a fraud. In the short term this may see dental professionals working harder than necessary to make sure that nobody finds out the 'truth'. Longer term, this self-doubt may cause anxiety or depression.

Imposter syndrome thoughts often impact high-achieving individuals, with a failure to internalise accomplishments and persistent self-doubt or fear of being exposed as a fraud being characteristic. Looking at the media, this type of thinking is often displayed in movies or TV; for example, the character of Betty in *Ugly Betty*, Andrea in *The Devil Wears Prada*, Remy in *Ratatouille,* and Bridget in the *Bridget Jones* franchise. Just as it is conveyed in the movies, the research shows that imposter syndrome is more common in marginalised groups, such as women and ethnic minorities. Individual factors play a role – such as low self-esteem – as do external factors, such as the toxic environment seen at *Runway* magazine in *The Devil Wears Prada*.

Imposter Syndrome Impacts Our Thoughts, Feelings, and Actions
Thoughts: Focused on competency, fear of failure, fear of being good enough or having fooled everyone to get to your position **Feelings:** Anxiety, low mood, depressive feelings **Actions:** Impacts professional progression as individuals may not put themselves forward for certain positions or upskilling, avoid delegation due to fear of appearing incompetent, withdraw, or disengage at work.

In general, imposter syndrome is associated with increased stress and burn-out and decreased job performance (Bravata et al. 2020). It also co-exists with depression, anxiety, and low self-esteem. Amongst medical professionals, imposter syndrome is more common in female medical students but also seen in males (Freeman and Peisah 2021). Experienced doctors also are affected (LaDonna et al. 2018). It can impact career progression, leadership, and mental health. Amongst nurses, as they progress, so does the incidence of imposter syndrome (John 2019), with difficulty in delegation common due to fear of being found out as incompetent.

Although there is limited research in dentistry on imposter syndrome, a study put forward an online module for 120 first-year dental students to help them cope with imposter syndrome (Metz et al. 2020). The authors reported that this online training module did improve awareness of imposter syndrome and help high-achieving students to cope.

Using Table 5.2, which details the different strategies we can employ, here are five ways dental professionals can manage imposter syndrome:

Mindful self-compassion: We can use Kristin Neff's (2003) three-step approach to provide us comfort whilst experiencing imposter syndrome thoughts.

1) Use mindfulness to notice the imposter syndrome thought and say to yourself: 'I notice I am having a thought. . .' (e.g. 'I notice I am having a thought that I am not good enough'). Labelling our thoughts helps us to create distance from thoughts and gives us greater perspective.

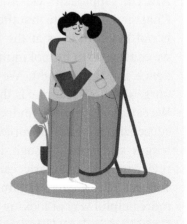

2) Remind yourself that you are not alone in experiencing negative thoughts. Remembering that we are all connected by tough experiences reminds us that we are not being singled out.

3) Notice where you experience the thought in your body. Soothe yourself with loving words or a soothing touch, such as squeezing your arm and saying 'I'm so sorry you are experiencing these thoughts. It's not nice to hear. I know you can do this and I believe in you'.

- **Acceptance:** We can use the 'weather analogy', where we remind ourselves that thoughts come and go. This helps us accept the experience, rather than to resist the thought, and also helps us to move through the emotion quicker. Alternatively, diffusion is a technique from acceptance and commitment therapy that gives us a way to stop fusing, or buying into the story of our thoughts. We can do this in several ways, such as using humour by saying the thoughts in a funny way, imagining the thought as a funny tag line on a newspaper, or singing the thought as a nursery rhyme.

- **CBT:** We can dispute the imposter syndrome thought through using the ABCDE approach we discuss in Chapter 8. If we note that the thought is not helpful for us at the moment, we can dispute it by looking at the evidence for the thought. We can ask ourselves, how accurate is this thought? What is a more realistic version? We can counteract the underlying fear of failure by reflecting on all of our successes and times at work where we managed to overcome similar challenges and grew through them. Keeping a 'compliments folder' and reviewing this regularly can also help to create a more positive self-concept. We can also reframe the thought by asking ourselves, what is a more helpful way of looking at this?

- **Growth mindset:** Using growth mindset can help us to build a more positive inner voice that focuses on progress, not outcomes or perfection.

Growth mindset is an essential component when we are learning and upskilling as dental professionals. We may do this through seeking a mentor and asking for feedback, celebrating our wins, using self-compassion, and remembering that our brains are neuroplastic and can change no matter what age. Alternatively, we may use positive growth mindset mantras. These are short, positive statements we repeat to help develop growth mindset, such as 'I worked hard at this', 'I embrace my success', 'I am creative and capable', or 'With every obstacle, I keep growing and getting better'. We can grow positive inner language by using Carol Dweck's three-step process (2006):

1) Recognising your fixed mindset inner dialogue (such as 'If I avoid challenges, others won't doubt me')
2) Recognising that mindset is a choice by thinking to yourself that you can shift your mindset with practice
3) Practising a growth mindset approach, for example, saying to yourself 'I focus on effort' or 'If I fail, I learn'.

- **Strengths:** Working out our character strengths by reflecting on them or using profilers, such as the free VIA survey on strengths (http://viacharacter.org), helps to remind us of our unique positive qualities. This is great for helping us navigate challenges, such as starting a new job, as well as upskilling.

In the following worksheets, we focus on how to use psychological strategies in relation to specific emotions and differing dental scenarios:

- Anxiety during a new dental procedure
- Feeling emotionally drained
- Feeling overwhelmed
- Feeling angry
- Having a low mood.

In the final section of this chapter, try these mind exercises to start exercising your resilience and well-being muscles. Each exercise guides you through a different dental scenario. As with all well-being tools, the key is to experiment and find out which tool works the best for you.

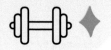

Tackling Anxiety At Work

1.   **Imagine you are just about to start a new clinical procedure.** You have recently upskilled, and this is one of the first times you are doing this procedure, such as a molar root canal, short-term orthodontics, or composite bonding. You notice fear and anxiety bubbling up. You wonder if you can do this. Your thoughts become very self-critical; you feel like you're not good enough. Select mind tools from the mind gym menu that can help you, in the moment, as you are with your patient.

2.   **Let's go through a few of the mind tools for anxiety in more detail.** If you selected the mindfulness and acceptance tools, what could you say to help soothe yourself in the moment? For example; 'Hello there, self-criticism! There you are. You come and go' or 'It's alright to be anxious, just let it be, it will go away'. Another example may be taking a deep breath.

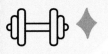

3. **Let's explore the self-compassion tool.** What loving, kind things can you say to yourself in the moment? For example, 'I'm so sorry you are feeling anxious right now. I know you will keep getting better with time, and I'm here for you every step of the way. I believe in you'. What non-verbal gestures can you do? An example may be trying a soothing physical gesture.

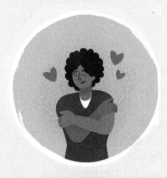

4. **Let's explore the cognitive reappraisal tool.** What could you say in the moment to help yourself reframe the situation in a more helpful way? For example, 'A more helpful way of looking at this situation is that I'm learning something new and that's tough, but with time and practice, I will get better and more comfortable'.

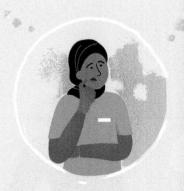

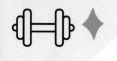

Managing Compassionate Care Challenges

Caring for our patients goes beyond just the management of their teeth. It is holistic care. We often see our patients suffering. It may be a newly diagnosed mental health condition, the loss of a partner, or a cancer diagnosis. This makes us particularly at risk of burnout and compassion fatigue. In this example, we explore ways to use mind tools during moments we notice feeling our energy levels drained as a result of our empathetic bonds with our patients.

1. **Imagine your long-standing patient comes in to her examination appointment after trauma to her arm, after an accident.** This is a patient you have been seeing for years and have developed a good relationship with. She can no longer feel any sensation on her arm due to this accident, and she is understandably very distraught. She tells you she is not feeling very well emotionally. You go through options of referral to GP and other professional services that can support her during this time. After your patient leaves, you notice feeling very drained emotionally. Which mind tools can you select to help you in this moment?

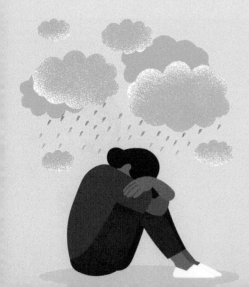

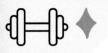

Managing Compassionate
Care Challenges

2. **Let's go through the self-compassion tool.** What words of kindness can you say to yourself in response to the difficult emotions you are feeling? Use the same language you would to a good friend you care about, for example, 'I know you feel so sad for your patient and to see her suffering. You didn't cause her suffering and you have helped the best you can. I'm here to support you.' What non-verbal gestures can you provide to help soothe you in the moment – for example, squeezing your arm or hand?

3. **Let's explore the talking tool next.** List people you can talk to that can help you in this moment; for example, speaking to my nurse, practice manager, and so forth.

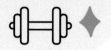

Overcoming Overwhelm

1. **Imagine you feel under pressure to complete targets.** You feel overwhelmed and stressed. These may be university quotas, UDA targets, or financial targets from your practice. Select mind tools from the mind gym menu that can help you, in the moment.

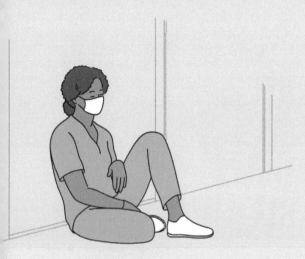

2. **Let's explore the problem-solving tool in more depth.** Brainstorm all possible solutions and write them down. Be creative. Nothing is off the table.

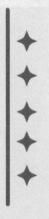

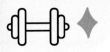

3. **Evaluate the pros and cons of each option.** Give each option a score out of 10. Once you've completed this exercise, you'll be able to problem solve the next time you have a situation that is within your control.

Option	Pro	Cons	Score/10

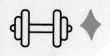

Noting Low Mood

1. **Imagine you are feeling sad and you notice your mood is low.** It's the first day you've noticed this feeling. Nothing bad has happened, but you just don't feel your 'regular' self. Which mind tools can you select to help you?

2. **Let's go through the pleasure and mastery tool to begin with.** Write down a list of things that give you pleasure – for example, talking to friends, watching Netflix, playing table tennis. Next write a list that gives you a sense of achievement (mastery). This second list can just be things you have to do but find hard – for example, chores, getting out of bed in the morning when you don't want to. You can then plan your day with a mixture of pleasure and mastery.

Pleasure	Mastery

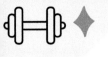

De-escalating Anger

1. **Let's explore the assertiveness tool next.** Write down a potential direct yet professional response to the patient; for example, 'I understand you are feeling frustrated, and I can tell you really want to save this tooth. I am happy to refer you for a second opinion to a specialist to discuss this further'.

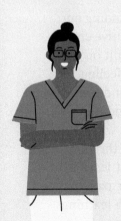

Summary

- Emotional intelligence is the ability to monitor our own and others' feelings and emotions, to discriminate among them and use this information as a guide to our own thinking and actions.
- Benefits of high EI for dental professionals include greater resilience and well-being; better quality of care to patients; greater career satisfaction; improved leadership, teamwork, and communication; and increased empathy.
- We can do this through understanding our emotional triggers, going with a curious attitude, increasing our emotional literacy, and accepting that no emotion is good or bad.
- Positive emotions have a broadening effect.
- Personality also impacts our experience of emotion.
- Strategies that can help build greater EI include mindfulness, self-compassion, cognitive reappraisal, exposure, problem solving, and physical exercise.

 The View From Here

The 'E' of PERLE spotlights emotional intelligence: that is, understanding our emotions, regulating our emotions, and harnessing the power of positive emotions. It is unsurprising that greater resilience and well-being is built on the foundation of understanding these emotions. To know how we are feeling, in our mind and body, and to be able to downregulate is a massively underrated but important mind tool. Whether we choose self-compassion, mindfulness, cognitive reappraisal, exposure, or acceptance at trigger points with our patients and at home, EI has tremendous benefits in helping us to thrive. In many ways, educating ourselves on emotional intelligence is about learning how we can show up better for ourselves, our loved ones, and our patients. These skills truly impact every aspect of our lives. We could do with learning these tools very early on, from childhood. Interestingly, school curricula are integrating lessons on understanding emotions, from labelling what we are feeling to learning about both mindfulness and compassion. Similarly, undergraduate curricula need a desperate upgrade.

A word on experimenting with these mind tools: be patient with yourself. We do not judge a seed for trying to become a flower. We do not care how long it takes to bloom or which direction it decides to grow. We simply admire the fact that it grows at all. We are mystified by it. Keeping self-compassion close by your side, allow your journey to harnessing your emotions unfold, with kindness and love towards yourself.

References

Aldao, A., Nolen-Hoeksema, S., and Schweizer, S. (2010). Emotion-regulation strategies across psychopathology: a meta-analytic review. *Clinical Psychology Review* 30 (2): 217–237. https://doi.org/10.1016/j.cpr.2009.11.004.

Beck, J.S. (1964). *Cognitive Therapy: Basics and Beyond*. New York: Guildford Press.

Bravata, D.M., Watts, S.A., Keefer, A.L. et al. (2020). Prevalence, predictors, and treatment of impostor syndrome: a systematic review. *Journal of General Internal Medicine* 35: 1252–1275. https://doi.org/10.1007/s11606-019-05364-1.

Broderick, P.C. (2005). Mindfulness and coping with dysphoric mood: contrasts with rumination and distraction. *Cognitive Therapy and Research* 29 (5): 501–510.

Costa, P.T. and McRae, R.R. (1980). Influence of extraversion and neuroticism on subjective well-being: happy and unhappy people. *Journal of Personality and Social Psychology* 38: 668–678.

Costa, P.T. and McRae, R.R. (1992). The five-factor model of personality and its relevance to personality disorders. *Journal of Personality Disorders* 6 (4): 343–359.

Cuijpers, P., van Straten, A., and Warmerdam, L. (2007). Behavioral activation treatments of depression: a meta-analysis. *Clinical Psychology Review* 27 (3): 318–326. https://doi.org/10.1016/j.cpr.2006.11.001.

Dweck, C.S. (2006). *Mindset: The New Psychology of Success*. New York: Random House.

Ekman, P. (2003). Darwin, deception, and facial expression. In: *Emotions Inside Out: 130 Years After Darwin's 'The Expression of the Emotions in Man and Animals'* (ed. P. Ekman, J.J. Campos, R.J. Davidson and F.B.M. de Waal), 205–221. New York: New York Academy of Sciences.

Ellis, A. (1957). Rational psychotherapy and individual psychology. *Journal of Individual Psychology 13*: 38–44.

Ford, B.Q., Lam, P., John, O.P., and Mauss, I.B. (2017). The psychological health benefits of accepting negative emotions and thoughts: laboratory, diary, and longitudinal evidence. *Journal of Personality and Social Psychology* (6): 115, 1075–1092. Advance online publication. https://doi.org/10.1037/pspp0000157.

Fredrickson, B.L. (2001). The role of positive emotions in positive psychology: the broaden-and-build theory of positive emotions. *The American Psychologist* 56 (3): 218–226. https://doi.org/10.1037//0003-066x.56.3.218.

Fredrickson, B.L. (2004). The broaden-and-build theory of positive emotions. *Philosophical Transactions of the Royal Society B* 359 (1449): 1367–1378.

Fredrickson, B.L. (2009). *Positivity: Groundbreaking Research Reveals How to Embrace the Hidden Strength of Positive Emotions, Overcome Negativity, and Thrive*. Crown Publishers/Random House.

Fredrickson, B.L. and Levenson, R.W. (1998). Positive emotions speed recovery from the cardiovascular sequelae of negative emotions. *Cognition and Emotion* 12 (2): 191–220. https://doi.org/10.1080/026999398379718.

Freeman, J. and Peisah, C. (2021). Imposter syndrome in doctors beyond training: a narrative review. *Australasian Psychiatry* 30 (1): 49–54. https://doi.org/10.1177/10398562211036121.

Galante, J., Dufour, G., Vainre, M. et al. (2018). A mindfulness-based intervention to increase resilience to stress in university students (the Mindful Student Study): a pragmatic randomised controlled trial. *Lancet Public Health* 3 (2): e72–e81. https://doi.org/10.1016/S2468-2667(17)30231-1.

Gilbert, P. and Procter, S. (2006). Compassionate mind training for people with high shame and self-criticism: overview and pilot study of a group therapy approach. *Clinical Psychology & Psychotherapy* 13: 353–379.

Gross, J.J. (1998). The emerging field of emotion regulation: an integrative review. *Review of General Psychology* 2 (3): 271–299. https://doi.org/10.1037/1089-2680.2.3.271.

Isen, A.M., Rosenzweig, A.S., and Young, M.J. (1991). The influence of positive affect on clinical problem solving. *Medical Decision Making* 11 (3): 221–227.

Jacobson, N.S., Dobson, K.S., Truax, P.A. et al. (1996). A component analysis of cognitive-behavioral treatment for depression. *Journal of Consulting and Clinical Psychology* 64 (2): 295–304. https://doi.org/10.1037/0022-006X.64.2.295.

John, S. (2019). Imposter syndrome: why some of us doubt our competence. *Nursing Times [online]* 115 (2): 23–24.

LaDonna, K.A., Ginsburg, S., and Watling, C. (2018). 'Rising to the level of your incompetence': what physicians' self-assessment of their performance reveals about the imposter syndrome in medicine. *Academic Medicine* 93 (5): 763–768. https://doi.org/10.1097/ACM.0000000000002046.

Leary, M.R., Tate, E.B., Adams, C.E. et al. (2007). Self-compassion and reactions to unpleasant self-relevant events: the implications of treating oneself kindly. *Journal of Personality and Social Psychology* 92 (5): 887–904. https://doi.org/1 0.1037/0022-3514.92.5.887.

Mayer, J.D. and Salovey, P. (2007). *Mayer–Salovey–Caruso emotional intelligence test*. Toronto: Multi-Health Systems Incorporated.

Mendolia, M. and Kleck, R.E. (1993). Effects of talking about a stressful event on arousal: does what we talk about make a difference? *Journal of Personality and Social Psychology* 64 (2): 283–292. https://doi.org/10.1037/0022-3514.64.2.283.

Metz, C., Ballard, E., and Metz, M. (2020). The stress of success: an online module to help first-year dental students cope with the impostor phenomenon. *Journal of Dental Education* 84 (9): 1016–1024.

Najmi, S., Amir, N., Frosio, K., and Ayers, C. (2014). The effects of cognitive load on attention control in subclinical anxiety and generalized anxiety disorder. *Cognition & Emotion* 29: 1–14. https://doi.org/10.1080/02699931.2014.975188.

Neff, K. (2003). Self-compassion: an alternative conceptualization of a healthy attitude toward oneself. *Self and Identity* 2 (2): 85–101.

Nolen-Hoeksema, S. and Morrow, J. (1993). Effects of rumination and distraction on naturally occurring depressed mood. *Cognition and Emotion* 7 (6): 561–570. https://doi.org/10.1080/02699939308409206.

Salovey, P. and Mayer, J.D. (1990). Emotional intelligence. *Imagination, Cognition and Personality* 9 (3): 185–211.

Sher, K.J. and Grekin, E.R. (2007). Alcohol and affect regulation. In: *Handbook of Emotion Regulation* (ed. J.J. Gross), 560–580. Guilford Press.

Shiota, M.N., Keltner, D., and John, O.P. (2006). Positive emotion dispositions differentially associated with big five personality and attachment style. *Journal of Positive Psychology* 1 (2): 61–71.

Sloan, T. and Telch, M.J. (2002). The effects of safety-seeking behavior and guided threat reappraisal on fear reduction during exposure: an experimental investigation. *Behaviour Research and Therapy* 40 (3): 235–251. https://doi. org/10.1016/S0005-7967(01)00007-9.

Stathopoulou, G., Powers, M.B., Berry, A.C. et al. (2006). Exercise interventions for mental health: a quantitative and qualitative review. *Clinical Psychology: Science and Practice* 13 (2): 179–193.

6

Emotional Intelligence – Using Mindfulness

CHAPTER OVERVIEW

- Understanding what mindfulness is
- Benefits of mindfulness for dental professionals
- Measure your mindfulness levels
- Neuroscience of mindfulness
- Mindfulness research
- Mindfulness and emotions
- Applying mindfulness.

> *The best way to capture moments is to pay attention. This is how we cultivate mindfulness. Mindfulness means being awake. It means knowing what you are doing.*
>
> —Jon Kabat-Zinn, mindfulness teacher, professor, author, and creator of the Mindfulness-Based Stress Reduction programme

Defined as paying attention to the present moment, with non-judgment, mindfulness is our ability to know what is in our heads at any given moment, without getting lost in the story of our thoughts. Our mind is constant chatter of anxious thoughts about the future or thoughts ruminating about the past. Mindfulness allows us to react with our emotions and thoughts with kindness, equanimity, and intelligence, so we aren't jerked around by those emotions and thoughts. This powerful tool also helps us hone all three components of emotional intelligence: self-awareness, emotional regulation, and fostering positive emotions.

To be a mindful dental professional means consciously cultivating the nine attitudes of mindfulness: non-judging, gratitude, patience, a beginner's mind, trust, non-striving, acceptance, letting go, and generosity (Kabat-Zinn 1990). And just like any muscle of the body, mindfulness can be trained and strengthened, and no matter what your starting point is, you can become more mindful tomorrow. In this chapter, we explore in depth how in dentistry we can infuse mindfulness at work and outside the clinic, reaping benefits for ourselves, the

Resilience and Well-being for Dental Professionals, First Edition. Mahrukh Khwaja.
© 2023 John Wiley & Sons Ltd. Published 2023 by John Wiley & Sons Ltd.
Companion website: www.wiley.com/go/khwaja-resilience-dentistry

dental team, and our patients and have downstream impacts on all of our wider relationships.

The experience of being on a rollercoaster is very different to observing a rollercoaster from a distance; similarly, mindfulness can give us distance to zoom out and gain perspective. Our minds are a constant chatter of thoughts of the past or future. When we are in the role of mindful observer, we have space to choose our words and actions rather than being reactive. We can step off the rollercoaster. We start noticing the beautiful details of our lives. Far from just a pain reliever, mindfulness is at its core an awakening of the senses. It is moving from autopilot mode, where we are doing things mindlessly, to being fully engaged with our reality.

Since anxiety and negative emotions are uncomfortable, we may have developed strategies to keep anxiety at bay. We try to control our emotions by resisting the negative emotions. This could be through the following strategies:

- **Bottling worries**: This takes a great deal of effort and can be very draining. It also brings an additional worry – that you will not be able to keep your emotions in.
- **Distracting yourself:** This prolongs the underlying problem and also may lead to other unhelpful coping strategies, such as excessive drinking, comfort eating, or scrolling on social media for prolonged periods of time.
- **Toxic positivity:** This is a belief that no matter how difficult the situation is, you should maintain a positive mindset. Toxic positivity can make people feel under pressure to pretend to be happy even if they are struggling. This is a harmful strategy, as it can lead to ignoring serious problems, a sense of isolation or stigma, and low self-esteem.

However, none of these strategies are likely to succeed, because when we avoid feeling and processing our emotions, those emotions amplify and may cause us to feel disconnected from ourselves or implode at unexpected times. Mindfulness involves acceptance rather than control.

A Self-Awareness Exercise: What's My Internal Weather?

In many ways, our emotions are like the weather. Clouds float away and rain stops. The weather does not stay the same forever. Similarly, our emotions and thoughts come and go. Are you feeling great, like a clear sunny day? Or grumpy, like a sky full of black clouds? Thinking of our emotions and thoughts in this way can help us gain a little objectivity and stay with them longer, rather than pushing them away. When we better understand our inner world, we can engage with it with greater curiosity and confidence. We can say to ourselves; 'I'm just feeling stormy, today. I'll feel better soon'.

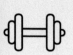

What's My Internal Weather?

Here is a mindful check-in to help you become more aware of your emotions.

1. Take a moment for yourself to take three deep breaths.
2. Ask yourself, 'What's my inner weather?' If you feel calm and happy, maybe that's a sunny day. Or if you're upset, maybe you feel like a stormy ocean. If you just let it be, and be a little curious about it, it will move along or change. Write this weather report on the clouds below.
3. Do this exercise at different points of the day. Reflect on how your 'weather' changes.

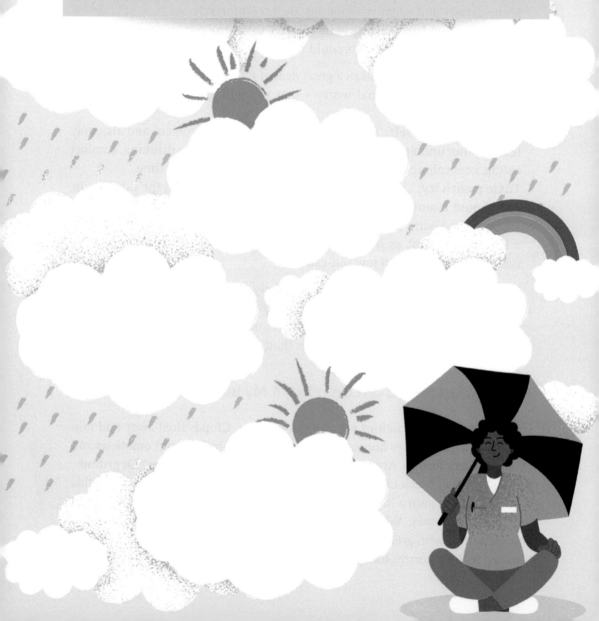

What's My Internal Weather?

Myth versus Fact

There are numerous myths around mindfulness that can be obstacles to us engaging with this practice. Following are the four most common myths I find when teaching mindfulness to dental professionals.

Myth 1: Mindfulness Is a Religious Practice

Although mindfulness gets its roots from several religions, namely Buddhism, mindfulness is in fact a secular practice that involves no religious chanting. It was brought over by American professor Jon Kabat-Zinn in 1979 as a way to help a very stressed population. He was inspired to formulate the Mindfulness-Based Stress Reduction programme after attending a talk by author Philip Kapleau, which introduced Kabat-Zinn to the concepts of mindfulness. Mindfulness focuses on breathing as a way of paying attention to the present moment.

Myth 2: Mindfulness Involves Not Having Thoughts

A common misconception of mindfulness is that this practice involves getting rid of thoughts. This is simply not possible, as our brains have a natural tendency to wander, and far from the practice of mindfulness. The mindfulness process involves paying attention to our breath, noticing our mind wander, and gently nudging our attention back to the breath with kind compassion.

Myth 3: Mindfulness Is the Same as Meditation

Mindfulness incorporates a wide range of activities, from meditations to mindful eating, mindful listening, and mindful movement. We can also apply mindfulness to every aspect of our lives, such as when we are with our patients, in a queue or driving to work, or brushing our teeth. With mindfulness, we are asking ourselves to pay attention to the present moment. Meditation, on the other hand, involves sitting down, often closing our eyes, and focusing our full attention inwards.

Myth 4: Mindfulness Can Only Be Practised in a Quiet Space

The wonderful aspect of mindfulness, specifically for busy dental professionals, is that it can be practised throughout our day, whatever the noise levels are, through integrating micro-moments of mindfulness. This could be, for example, when we are drinking a cup of tea in the morning and taking three mindful breaths. Alternatively, it could be when we are at work, listening mindfully to our patients. We can also integrate mindfulness meditations, but this does not necessarily mean we need a quiet space to commit to it.

Measure Your Well-being: Mindfulness

How mindful are you? Measure your current level of mindfulness using the Five Facet Mindfulness Questionnaire (FFMQ) (adapted from Bohlmeijer et al. 2011) below.

For each statement, indicate the response that best applies to you in the past week, using the following scale.

Almost never		Sometimes true		Almost always
1	2	3	4	5

Observing

___1. I pay attention to physical experiences, such as the wind in my hair or sun on my face.

___2. Generally, I pay attention to sounds, such as clocks ticking, birds chirping, or cars passing by.

___3. I notice the smell and aromas of things.

___4. I notice the visual elements in art or nature, such as colours, shapes, textures, or patterns of light and shadow.

Describing

___5. I'm good at finding the words to describe my feelings.

___6. I can easily put my beliefs, opinions, and expectations into words.

___7. Even when I'm feeling terribly upset, I can find a way to put it into words.

___8. It's hard for me to find the words to describe how I am feeling.

___9. When I feel something in my body, it's hard for me to find the right words to describe it.

Acting with awareness

___10. I find a way to stay focused on what is happening in the present moment.

___11. It seems I am 'running on automatic' without much awareness of what I'm doing.

___12. I rush through activities without being really attentive to them.

___13. I do jobs or tasks automatically without being aware of what I'm doing.

___14. I find myself doing things without paying attention.

Measure Your Well-being: Mindfulness

For each statement, indicate the response that best applies to you in the past week, using the following scale.

Almost never		Sometimes true		Almost always
1	2	3	4	5

Nonjudging of inner experience
___15. I tell myself that I shouldn't be feeling the way I'm feeling.
___16. I make judgments about whether my thoughts are good or bad.
___17. I tell myself I shouldn't be thinking the way I'm thinking.
___18. I think some of my emotions are bad or inappropriate and I should not feel them.
___19. I disapprove of myself when I have illogical ideas.

Nonreactivity to inner experience
___20. I watch my feelings without getting carried away by them.
___21. When I have distressing thoughts, I don't let myself be carried away by them.
___22. When I have distressing thoughts, I feel calm soon after.
___23. Usually when I have distressing thoughts, I can just notice them without reacting.
___24. When I have distressing thoughts, I just notice them and let them go.

Scoring

To get the overall score, sum the item scores and divide by 24. Scores range between 1 and 5. Higher scores indicate greater mindfulness.

A Superpower in Dentistry

Practising mindfulness as dental professionals allows us to create space in our minds for joy, relaxation, peace, inspiration, ideas, creativity, and confidence to thrive in the workplace and outside. We can think of mindfulness as a tool to help us pay attention, with kindness, to the here and now. It can give us a whole novel approach to life that actively invites more positive emotions: self-compassion, gratitude, curiosity, and acceptance.

There are numerous psychological, physical, and psychosocial benefits of practising mindfulness reported in the literature. These include an increase in positive well-being states; for example, life satisfaction, engagement with health-related behaviours, better sleep, improved thinking and memory, and a reduction in negative well-being states, such as burnout and compassion fatigue. Mindfulness also helps our interpersonal relationships by nurturing our listening skills and our ability to empathise with our patients and loved ones.

Looking back at Chapter 1, and thinking about the mental health continuum, mindfulness is a protective factor that can boost our resilience levels and our mental well-being.

Neuroscience of Mindfulness

Neuroscience research has also caught up with the increasing belief that mindfulness is beneficial. These studies validate over and over that mindfulness indeed can change the brain structure in positive ways.

Let us hone into the specific changes the brain makes in response to mindfulness practice:

- **Amygdala:** Mindfulness may reduce the grey matter of our amygdala. The functional connections between the amygdala and pre-frontal cortex are also strengthened. This allows for less reactivity when it comes to our stress triggers.
- **Hippocampus:** Mindfulness improves the work of the hippocampus, our 'librarian', which strengthens our recall and storage for memories and important information.
- **Pre-frontal cortex:** The grey matter of this region of the brain can increase with mindfulness practice (Gotink et al. 2016). This results in enhancing our executive function abilities, such as memory, attention, planning, and problem solving.
- **Default mode network (DMN):** Decreased activation of the DMN is associated with excessive worrying and commonly found in depression or

anxiety. Mindfulness switches on the alternative brain network, known as the task positive network. It is associated with 'flow state', and much of the time, we are happier when we are using this network.

- **Anterior cingulate cortex**: Increased grey matter changes in this region allow for more thinking flexibility.

Clough and colleagues reported that relaxation modalities, such as mindfulness-based interventions (MBIs), reduced physician stress, burnout, psychological distress, and self-compassion (Clough et al. 2017; Krasner et al. 2009; Ospina-Kammerer and Figley 2003; Shapiro et al. 1998). MBIs may help clinicians by fostering attitudes of acceptance, compassion, and non-judgment in addition to a new relationship with difficult emotions at work, such as observing anxiety without interaction during a stressful procedure.

Managing Our Energy and Emotions

The circumplex model of emotions (see Figure 6.1) (Russell 1980) describes different zones we experience, along an axis of high or low energy and negative or positive emotions. Understanding which zone we are currently in by regular mindful check-ins can help us better take care of our mental well-being by thinking of steps, if needed, that can shift us towards the recovery zone.

Survival zone: This is characterised by negative emotions and high energy. This zone is where many of us may find ourselves spending a lot of time, trying to meet the demands of patients and our personal lives.

Burnout zone: The burnout zone is characterised by low energy and negative emotions. Dental professionals early on in their careers may be at increased susceptibility to depersonalisation and work–life conflicts (see Chapter 1 for an in-depth look at burnout).

Recovery zone: This is characterised by low energy and positive emotions. Without recharging and carving out time for self-care, it is very difficult to reach the performance or thriving zone, where many leaders find they do their optimal work.

Performance zone: The performance zone is characterised by high energy and positive emotions. The performance zone, otherwise known as the thriving zone, is a zone where we feel engaged, connected, optimistic, and challenged but not to the point of being burnt out. This is often the zone where we are personally motivated to do great work and enjoy the process of doing so.

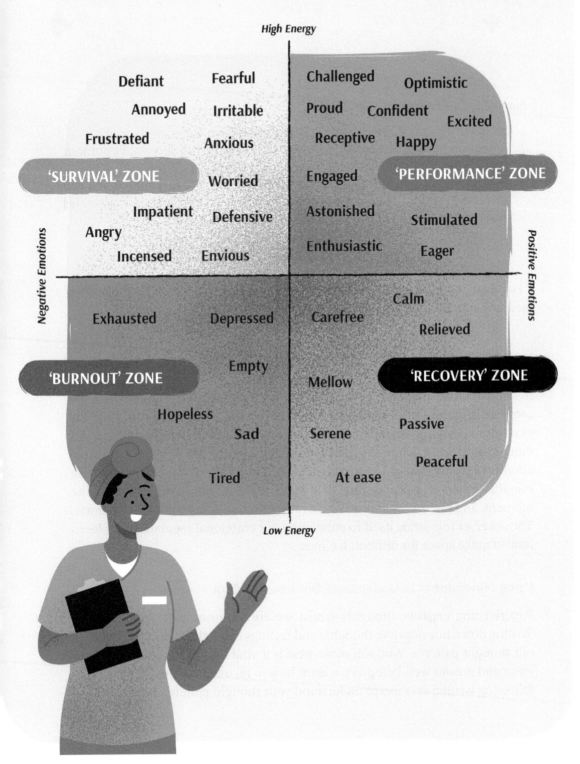

Figure 6.1   The circumplex model of emotions.

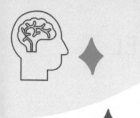

Think About It

For a guided meditation of the above exercise, see the *Burnout Recognition* meditation in the companion website.

Inner Critic versus Mindful Observer

In dentistry, treatments sometimes do not go according to plan. They may be complex in nature or communication with patients may be challenging; for example, managing anxious patients or patients with high expectations. An inner critical voice is one that mocks us for things not running smoothly. It is often mistakenly thought as a motivator but, in reality, it is detrimental. The mindful observer voice is one that stays present, non-judgmental of the moment, and reports what is going on rather than creating a negative rhetoric. The observer role lends itself to enhancing our emotional regulation. We learn how to make space for difficult feelings.

Using Mindfulness to Understand Our Inner Dialogue

Experiencing negative thoughts whilst we are with our patients is natural. Writing down our negative thoughts and feelings can help us become aware of our thought patterns. And self-awareness is a vital first step in building resilience and greater well-being as we learn how to regulate our emotions. Try the following writing exercise to understand your thought patterns better.

Negative Automatic Thoughts

1. Reflect on any negative thoughts or feelings you have during the day with patients. This could be during treatment or in anticipation of seeing a particular patient.
2. Write these down in the thought bubbles on the image below.
3. Try to write these thoughts with kindness and non-judgment. No emotion or thought is wrong.
4. How do you feel having written this down? Are you surprised by the content? Would you say any of these things to a friend?
5. Reflect on your responses. Think of how accurate the negative thoughts are. What's the evidence against this negative thought? Reflect on kind words you could use to soothe yourself in these moments.
6. Write down possible positive self-talk inner dialogue; for example, 'I'm not good enough' could be 'I am a work in progress. Each day I learn and improve. With time and effort, I can do this'.

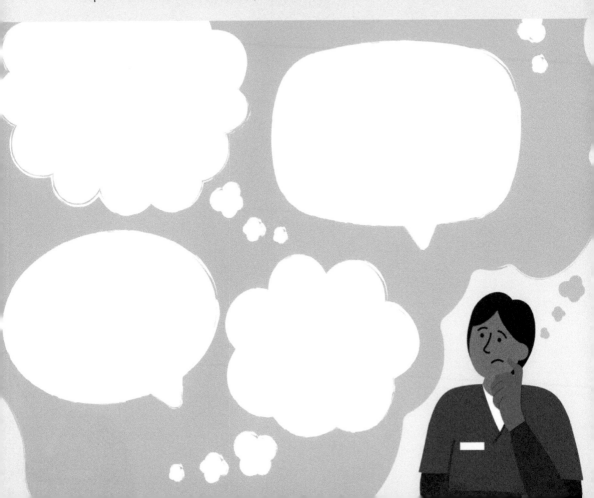

The Mindfulness Meditation Process

The process of mindfulness meditation is straightforward, but often many of us think we are doing it wrong, simply because our mind keeps wandering. It is very natural for one's mind to wander. Mindfulness meditation involves focusing in on our breath, noticing ourselves becoming distracted, and then with kindness and compassion gently nudging our attention back to the breath. It is this process of focus, distraction, and refocus that builds our muscles of resilience and self-compassion.

When you start practising mindfulness meditation for the first time, you may want to begin with meditations for 30 seconds to 1 minute. Build this up slowly to 5 minutes, then 10–20 minutes. The best way of creating a habit that sticks is ensuring you do start very small so that you can definitely achieve it! This then positively reinforces your habit and encourages you to keep going with it. You can also try stacking a mindfulness practice onto existing habits, such as going for a walk or reading a book. You may also want to try a mindfulness bell, which is an alarm to remind you, or use visual aids, such as a mindfulness cushion.

Mind Wandering and the Brain during Mindfulness

During mindfulness practice, it can be very frustrating when one's mind wanders. We may feel that we are not practising it right. However, do not despair! The human brain is hard wired for mind wandering! In fact, on average, 46.9% of our time we spend not paying attention! But why does the mind wander?

Our brain has two networks: the default mode network (DMN) and the task-positive network (TPN) (see Figure 6.2). The DMN is most active at rest, whereas

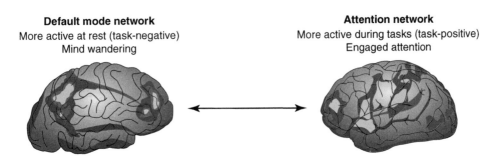

Default mode network
More active at rest (task-negative)
Mind wandering

Attention network
More active during tasks (task-positive)
Engaged attention

Figure 6.2   The two networks of the brain.

during mindfulness, we are engaging with the TPN. When we are focusing in on the breath during mindful practice, it can become unstimulating after a while – and hence our mind wanders. We are mostly thinking about ourselves; us in the past, us in the future, mostly problem solving or, if we are anxious, excessively chewing over a problem (rumination). Neuroscientists have discovered that the DMN state of mind wandering is associated with lower levels of happiness and increase in rumination, often a mind state linked with depression. During mindfulness, when we are fully engaging with the present, the DMN is less active, with the TPN on. We feel better!

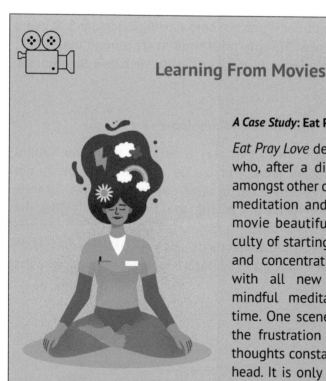

Learning From Movies

A Case Study: Eat Pray Love

Eat Pray Love describes the story of Liz, who, after a divorce, travels to India, amongst other countries, to learn about meditation and looking inwards. The movie beautifully captures the difficulty of starting a meditation practice and concentrating on the breath. As with all new habits, settling into mindful meditation can take some time. One scene effectively illustrates the frustration of Liz as she notices thoughts constantly popping up in her head. It is only when she accepts this mind-wandering quality of the brain that she is able to redirect her attention with kindness to her breath and focus on meditation. The good news is that there are several ways we can help ourselves stick with the practice of meditation! See the *Mindfulness Tips* below for some ideas to get you started.

Mindfulness Meditation Tips

- Mind wandering may present as sleepiness, boredom, restlessness, doubt, or aversion. A method of practising meditation whilst we experience the obstacles to mindfulness is to recognise and label the obstacle. Once we do this, we can mindfully accept the hindrance and bring gentle curiosity to it. We can consider how we feel it in our body and thoughts. Once we observe it as a fleeting process, we can sit with meditations without the judgment that we are doing it wrong.
- One effective way of being gentle on yourself when your mind wanders is to treat the brain like a toddler – with warmth, kindness, and compassion. Gently nudge your attention back to the breath.

Putting It into Practice

Mindfulness in the Clinic

As a dental professional struggling to find time to practise mindfulness, you will be pleased to know that mindfulness can indeed be practised at work! Try the next Mind-Flossing Exercise to integrate mindfulness throughout your clinical day (see *Mindfulness at Work*).

Body Scan

A mindfulness body scan is an exercise in which we bring awareness to all parts of our body, from the crown of our head to the tips of our toes. This exercise can be integrated into our morning routine. When we wake up, for example, we can do a quick body scan to check in and bring mindfulness to our next moments instead of reaching out for our phone. See the *Body Scan* meditation exercise and the companion website for a guided meditation.

Letting Go of Worries

A river can be a beautiful metaphor of life: we all have worries and obstacles, but we can learn to let go of them, just as the river ebbs and flows over rocks and plants. Try the river mindful meditation for letting go of worries (*Letting Go of Worries Meditation* exercise) and see the companion website for a guided meditation.

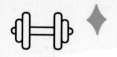

Mindfulness At Work

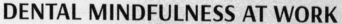
DENTAL MINDFULNESS AT WORK

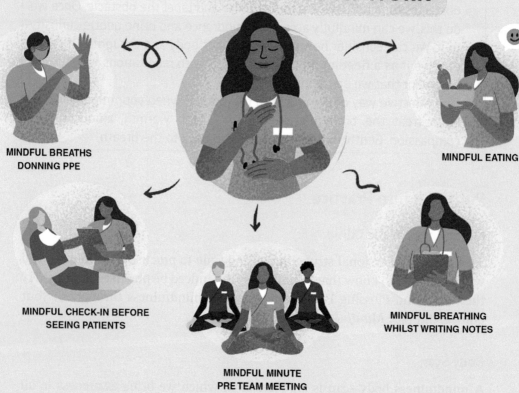

MINDFUL BREATHS
DONNING PPE

MINDFUL EATING

MINDFUL CHECK-IN BEFORE
SEEING PATIENTS

MINDFUL BREATHING
WHILST WRITING NOTES

MINDFUL MINUTE
PRE TEAM MEETING

- **Mindfulness breaths whilst donning/doffing PPE:** Slow down and take a couple of mindful breaths as you wear your PPE.

- **Mindful check-in before seeing each patient:** Ask yourself how you feel in your body, what emotions you are feeling, and whether you need a break before you bring your next patient into the surgery.

- **Mindful minute pre–team meeting:** Take a mindful minute as a team together before starting the agenda for a team meeting. This is a great way to settle yourself and bring back focus to a meeting.

- **Mindful breathing whilst writing notes.**

- **Mindfulness deep breaths during treatment:** For example, whilst administering local anaesthetic or waiting for impression material to set.

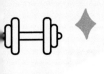

Body Scan

1

Set aside a time and place in your day where you can sit comfortably and you won't be distracted or disturbed.

2

Find a comfortable but attentive seated position, close your eyes, and bring your attention to your toes.

3

Working up from your toes, bring awareness to each body part in turn: your feet, ankles, calves, knees, etc. up to your head.

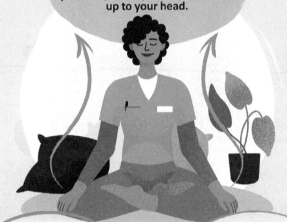

HEALTH BENEFITS:

- Reduced stress
- Decreased muscle tension
- Increased pain tolerance

WHY IT WORKS TO REDUCE STRESS:

Body scan meditations encourage self-awareness of sensations we might otherwise be ignoring.

1. Get in a comfortable position, either sitting down with your back supported or lying down. Close your eyes.

2. Bring your awareness to your breath. Notice how your breath feels with every inhale and exhale. Note the change in temperature and the sounds you make, as your chest rises and falls.

3. Now bring your attention to the toes. Note any discomfort here or tension. If you note this, bring comfort by stretching or soothing this area with another deep breath.

4. Go through each body part, from your ankles to your calves to your thighs and your stomach, until you have scanned every part of your body. You may want to imagine a warm light as you scan each body part in turn.

5. If you notice your mind wandering, do not worry. This is very natural. Gently nudge your attention back to your breath and continue until you reach the crown of your head.

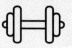

Letting Go of Worries Meditation

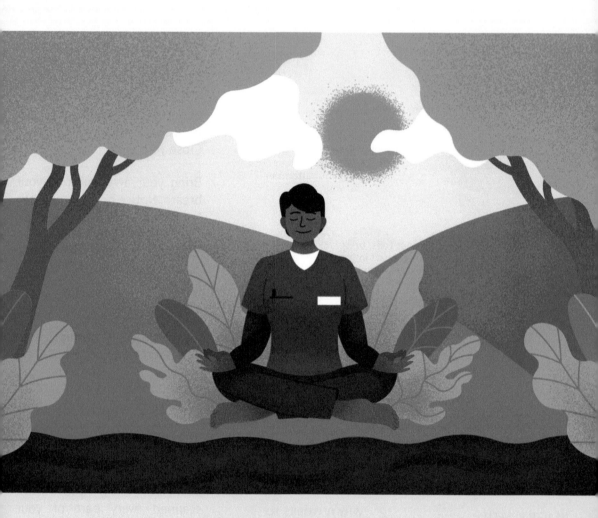

1. Start in a comfortable seated or lying down position, closing your eyes.
2. Imagine that you can see a river in front of you. Slowly walk towards the river until you're standing on the river bank.
3. Take a seat.
4. Note the landscape around the river. What sounds can you hear? What can you smell? What is the colour of the water? Does it run fast or slowly?
5. Place whatever is causing worry onto a leaf and into the water, watching your worry set off downstream.
6. Whenever a worry enters your head, that's fine. Allow it to enter and simply find a leaf to place it on and then set it off downstream.
7. When you're ready, slowly get up from the riverbank's edge and walk away from the river.
8. Slowly open your eyes.

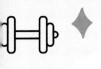

Zoom In

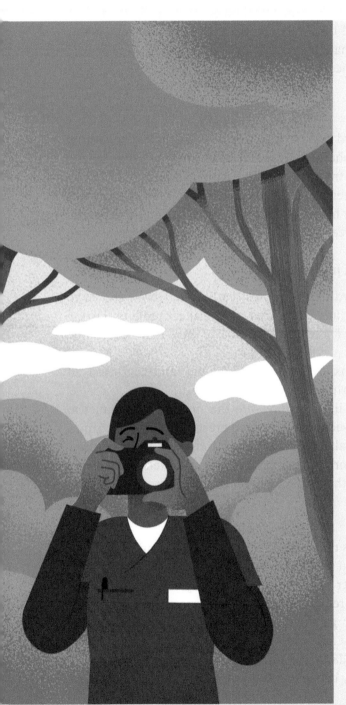

1. Head to a green space.

2. Before you take a photo, take a look around you. What are you looking at? Note the colours, textures, light, size, shapes, reflections, and angles.

3. Zoom into a colour or texture that captures your attention and explore this during your walk.

4. Remember to hone into the attitudes of mindfulness – non-judgment, curiosity, openness, and beginner's mind – as you take your photos.

Mindful Photography

Mindfulness, combined with creative pursuits, is one way to experience 'flow', otherwise known as being 'in the zone' and fully immersed in the activity we are doing so much that we lose all track of time. Being in flow has tremendous benefits for our well-being and happiness levels. Try this mindful nature walk to top up your levels of flow. See the *Zoom In* exercise.

Mindfulness Outdoors

Shinrin-yoku is a Japanese word that translates as 'forest bath'. Forest bathing is being in the forest atmosphere, fully immersed using our five senses. Although probably a very old tradition, it was first coined as a term in the 1980s by the Japanese Department of Forest and Fisheries. Forest bathing was developed in response to major health and stress problems from the Japanese urban population. There have been more than 30 years of scientific studies into the benefits of forest bathing.

There are numerous benefits, including:

- **Changes in immunity:** Two hours of forest bathing has been shown to increase NK cells in the body and expression of anticancer proteins, lasting up to 30 days (Li et al. 2007). These changes indicate there may be immune system effects.
- **Psychological benefits:** Anxiety, depression, fatigue, and confusion all reduced after forest bathing trips (Furuyashiki et al. 2019).
- **Blood pressure:** Reduction in blood pressure that may be an adjunct to blood pressure medication used to reduce blood pressure after only 15 minutes of forest therapy (Li et al. 2007). An overall reduction in blood pressure after one day of forest therapy, lasting up to five days after. This is likely due to increased activity of the parasympathetic nervous system inducing relaxation.
- **Decreased insomnia.**

There are three main theories that explain why nature is so important to us. One focuses on our reduction in stress (Attention Restoration Theory; Kaplan and Kaplan 1989) and the other two on our evolutionary bias towards green spaces. Humans have spent more than 99.99% of their time evolutionarily in a natural environment, and our genetics have adapted to nature. Since the Industrial Revolution, in the last 300 years we no longer spend as much time in nature, but our genes are still adapted to a natural environment.

Try the *Forest Bathing* activity below to discover the benefits of mindfulness outdoors for yourself.

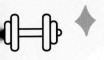

Forest Bathing

Here are six ways you can forest bathe, stimulating all five senses:

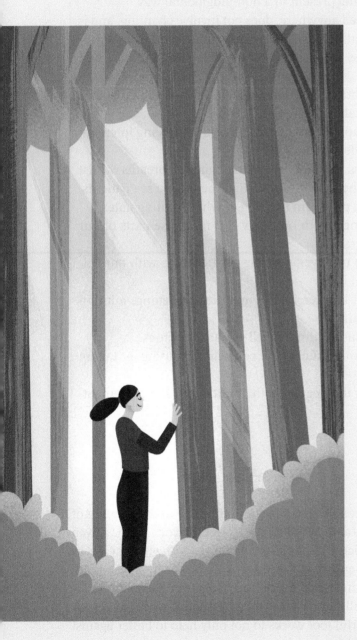

1. **See:** Lie down on the forest ground and look up at the sky. What do you see? Note the different colours, light and dark, textures, trees, animals, and movement in the forest.

2. **Touch:** Touch the mossy trees, the plants, twigs, branches. Note the different textures and temperatures.

3. **Smell:** Note the different smells. Take a leaf or plant or flower and breathe it in.

4. **Taste:** Some plants are edible, such as wild garlic. Have a taste.

5. **Hear:** Listen to the sounds of the forest, the birdsong, sway of the trees, the rustle of leaves, the sounds of insects, and the hum of the river stream.

6. **Slow down:** Have a seat and practice mindfulness in the forest. Tune into your breath and use the sounds of the forest to ground yourself back to the present moment.

For a range of guided meditations covering a range of positive psychology topics, from gratitude and optimism to strengths, values, and self-compassion, see the companion website.

Summary

- Mindfulness is a way of being present in a non-judgmental way.
- Mindfulness can be practised anywhere, does not involve chanting, and is not the same as mediation, although it does incorporate formal mediations.
- The benefits of mindfulness are vast: greater psychological, physical, and psychosocial health.
- Mindfulness impacts the brain; it reduces grey matter in the amygdala and increases the pre-frontal cortex.
- There is vast research to support mindfulness-based well-being interventions targeting medical professionals.
- We can apply mindfulness at work by taking mindful breaths whilst administering local anaesthetic, donning PPE, or before we see patients; or taking a mindful minute pre–team meeting or whilst writing notes.
- Body scans help us to connect with our body and recognise parts of our body that may be under stress.
- Mindful listening can help us develop strong relationships with our colleagues and in our personal lives.
- Mindfulness in nature can be exercised by mindful gardening, mindful nature walks, or forest bathing.
- Forest bathing encourages us to stimulate all of our five senses.
- Creative ways we can use mindfulness are colouring, painting, or taking photographs in nature.
- Mindful yoga is a great way to integrate both mindfulness and movement.

 The View From Here

Mindfulness has personally been the most useful tool in my understanding of my own emotions and thoughts and my emotional triggers at work and has given me a pathway to accepting difficult emotions or challenges with greater ease, as well as helping to increase my sense of engagement with the small, yet beautiful, details of my life. When teaching dental teams and dental professionals, mindfulness is well received, especially as a way to feel nourished at work during our busy clinical days. This wonderful tool works to not only help to buffer against dental stressors but also in creating a more meaningful life, because it encourages us to be present and take stock of all what we have to be grateful for.

The research amongst medical professionals on mindfulness-based interventions points to mindfulness having a real positive impact as preventative education. This has enormous implications regarding prevention for dental students and postgraduates, early on in their careers. As a potential protective factor when it comes to our mental well-being, mindfulness can be applied in so many creative ways. Whether we are practising mindfulness meditations or taking a couple of deep breaths whilst administering local anaesthetic to a patient, mindfulness can be integrated despite a busy schedule. It is in those little pockets of time, from waiting for the alginate impression to set or for your computer to load up every morning, that dental professionals can embrace the use of mindfulness to slow down, take stock of things we are grateful for, be engaged with the present, and show up at work, moment to moment.

References

Bohlmeijer, E., ten Klooster, P.M., Fledderus, M. et al. (2011). Psychometric properties of the Five Facet Mindfulness Questionnaire in depressed adults and development of a short form. *Assessment* 18 (3): 308–320.

Clough, B.A., March, S., Chan, R.J. et al. (2017). Psychosocial interventions for managing occupational stress and burnout among medical doctors: a systematic review. *Systematic Reviews* 6 (1): 1–19.

Furuyashiki, A., Tabuchi, K., Norikoshi, K. et al. (2019). A comparative study of the physiological and psychological effects of forest bathing (Shinrin-yoku) on working age people with and without depressive tendencies. *Environmental Health and Preventive Medicine* 24: 46. https://doi.org/10.1186/s12199-019-0800-1.

Gotink, R.A., Meijboom, R., Vernooij, M.W. et al. (2016). 8-week mindfulness based stress reduction induces brain changes similar to traditional long-term meditation practice – a systematic review. *Brain and Cognition* 108: 32–41. https://doi.org/10.1016/j.bandc.2016.07.001.

Kabat-Zinn, J. (1990). Full catastrophe living: Using the wisdom of your body and mind to face stress, pain and illness. New York, NY: Delacorte.

Kaplan, R. and Kaplan, S. (1989). *The Experience of Nature: A Psychological Perspective*. New York: Cambridge University Press.

Krasner, M.S., Epstein, R.M., Beckman, H. et al. (2009). Association of an educational program in mindful communication with burnout, empathy, and attitudes among primary care physicians. *JAMA* 302 (12): 1284–1293. https://doi.org/10.1001/jama.2009.1384.

Li, Q., Morimoto, K., Nakadai, A. et al. (2007). Forest bathing enhances human natural killer activity and expression of anti-cancer proteins. *International Journal of Immunopathology and Pharmacology* 3–8. https://doi.org/10.117 7/03946320070200S202.

Ospina-Kammerer, V. and Figley, C. (2003). An evaluation of the Respiratory One Method (ROM) in reducing emotional exhaustion among family physician residents. *International Journal of Emergency Mental Health* 5 (1): 29–32.

Russell, J.A. (1980). A circumplex model of affect. *Journal of Personality and Social Psychology* 39 (6): 1161–1178.

Shapiro, S.L., Schwartz, G.E., and Bonner, G. (1998). Effects of mindfulness-based stress reduction on medical and premedical students. *Journal of Behavioral Medicine* 21 (6): 581–599. https://doi.org/10.1023/a:1018700829825.

7

Emotional Intelligence – Fostering Self-compassion

CHAPTER OVERVIEW

- Benefits of self-compassion for dental professionals
- Relationship between perfectionism and self-compassion
- Measure your self-compassion levels
- Dispelling the myths
- Physiology of self-criticism and self-compassion
- Applying self-compassion at work and home.

> *Self-compassion is a way of emotionally recharging our batteries. Rather than becoming drained by helping others, self-compassion allows us to fill up our internal reserves, so we have more to give to those who need us.*
>
> —Kristin Neff, psychologist and professor at the University of Texas, researcher on mindful self-compassion

Self-compassion is another highly relevant and important tool in helping dental professionals become more emotionally intelligent. Wrapping up the EI section, in this chapter we delve deep into why self-compassion is essential in practising dentistry and how we can emotionally charge our batteries to keep giving to our patients.

As a dental professional, many of us chose our careers in dentistry because we feel compassion for others and want to help our patients feel better. We work hard to keep our patients well, but our own wellness can be sidelined. Chapter 1 delved into the high stressors that influence our mental well-being, the occupational hazards, and how personality traits, such as maladaptive perfectionism and a harsh inner critic, can push us beyond our limits and lead to psychological distress.

In this chapter, we will explore how to build resilience and greater psychological well-being through fostering self-compassion as clinicians. Treating patients without losing ourselves and enhancing our levels of compassion satisfaction – that is, the positive feelings we get from caring for our patients – is a lifelong journey. The journey starts with understanding the concept of self-compassion and the roots of perfectionism in us.

Resilience and Well-being for Dental Professionals, First Edition. Mahrukh Khwaja.
© 2023 John Wiley & Sons Ltd. Published 2023 by John Wiley & Sons Ltd.
Companion website: www.wiley.com/go/khwaja-resilience-dentistry

The problem with relying solely on self-care practices to manage our mental health is that it can often be difficult to find time. For example, we may not be able to take a timeout to go for a yoga session during a clinic when emotionally triggered during treatment with a patient. Self-compassion tools allow us to focus, in the moment, with patients and recalibrate so we can invite greater kindness, warmth, and support during those challenging moments of our day. Self-compassion provides us with the emotional resources needed to nurture ourselves. It is also a protective factor for caregivers, reducing the 'numbing out' effect of working closely with patients and minimising burnout and compassion fatigue.

A Radical Way of Relating to Ourselves

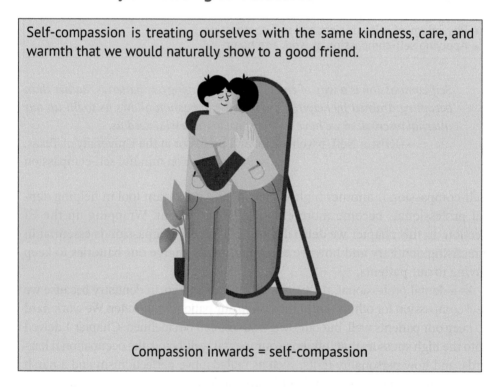

Self-compassion is treating ourselves with the same kindness, care, and warmth that we would naturally show to a good friend.

Compassion inwards = self-compassion

As a dental professional, showing compassion to our patients is one of our key personality traits that allow us to connect and build strong patient relationships. Self-compassion is compassion directed towards ourselves. It is a way of relating to ourselves with warm-heartedness and kindness in all moments, including those moments of suffering. It involves treating ourselves in a way we would treat a friend who is having a hard time – with generosity, gentleness, support, sympathy, and love. You could consider it almost as a radical approach as a healthcare professional, with the swapping of perfectionism and self-criticism with an approach that embraces our imperfections, soothes us when treatments fail or patients complain, and allows us to stay connected with the present, without getting stuck in negative thoughts about the past or swept up by anxious thoughts of the future.

Understanding the Perfectionism Trap: A Barrier to Self-compassion

Perfectionist traits are high amongst dental students and dental professionals. This comes as no surprise considering the emphasis of good grades in dental school and the high level of performance demanded working with patients. A recent study looking at 412 UK dental students reported high levels of perfectionism (35%), which was shown to be associated with maladaptive coping (avoidant coping strategies such as alcohol misuse or denial) and decreased mental well-being, specifically burnout, and psychological distress (Collin et al. 2020). Perfectionism in the research has been associated with decreased self-esteem and increase in depression and anxiety and unhelpful coping strategies (Grzegorek et al. 2004; Mehr and Adams 2016).

But what exactly is a perfectionist trait, and how does it present in dental professionals? A perfectionist trait is one where we set unreasonably high standards for ourselves and sometimes for others. It is the impossible quest to be perfect without flaws. At Stanford University, perfectionism is affectionately known as the Duck Syndrome – a duck appearing to glide calmly across the water, while beneath the surface, it frantically, relentlessly paddles.

The consequence of unrealistically high standards is that perfectionists are highly self-critical. Every flaw is scrutinised, ruminated upon, and used to self-flagellate. This inner critic may present as the internalised voice of our parents, teachers, or a bully. It may also originate from the media perpetuating that you are different, particularly in marginalised identity groups, such as groups excluded as a result of ethnicity, gender, identity, sexual orientation, and immigration status.

Further probing into perfectionist traits reveals a deep-rooted need to be liked, accepted, and loved. The underpinning belief beneath perfectionism is that achievement and performance determine our self-worth. There is often a fear of not being good enough. Perfection can be celebrated in society – for example, with successes of great athletes – and is often mistakenly confused with the pursuit of excellence. Anything less than being self-critical is an act of self-complacency. Individuals with high perfectionist traits strive to never make mistakes and are excruciatingly hard on themselves when they do.

It comes as no surprise that perfectionist traits do not lend to high levels of resilience. We do not easily dust ourselves from setbacks, and mistakes stick with us and damage our self-esteem. As such, perfectionism is a losing game. The unforgiving nature of perfectionism results in us feeling a lot worse rather than better. Perfectionism also denies the very nature of being human: perfectly imperfect.

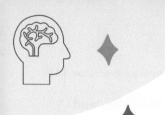

Think About It

The roots of perfectionistic traits originate in childhood, from growing up with unrealistic expectations from caretakers or from culture and media. In a better world, culture would endlessly draw to our attention to the first drafts and the hidden labours of the people behind the scenes. The challenge we have as adults is to uncover our own silent guides and update them so that we are not at the mercy of the perfectionism trap.

Perfectionism–Procrastination Loop

Do you catch yourself delaying or postponing getting important tasks done? Did you know that perfectionism trait and procrastination are linked? In the procrastination–perfection avoidance loop (see Figure 7.1), procrastination is

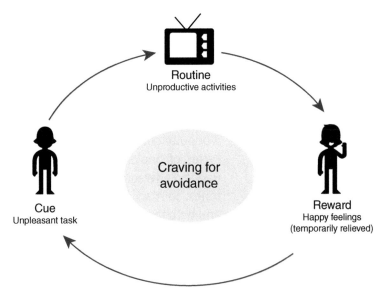

Figure 7.1 The procrastination–perfectionism avoidance loop.

not a case of poor time management or lack of motivation. Beneath the learnt habit of procrastination lie the same fears of the perfectionistic trait of not being good enough or failing. It is this fear that prevents us beginning altogether. The common thread in the habit of procrastination is that the important tasks that are being delayed are not seen as fun or are stressful. Thinking of completing the task creates thoughts of not being good enough and not meeting our high standards, and the emotions of anxiety, fear, and doubt creep in. This leads to the avoidance of the task to relieve ourselves from negative emotions caused by the negative thoughts, with alternative routine tasks taking priority, such as scrolling through social media. We feel a sense of reward when our negative emotions are temporarily reduced; however, soon enough our minds return to the task, and the avoidance loop continues!

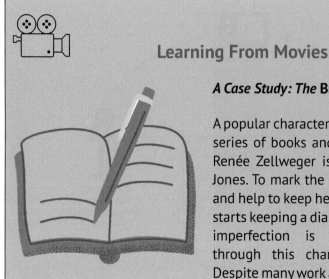

Learning From Movies

A Case Study: The Bridget Jones *Series*

A popular character from Helen Fielding's series of books and the movies starring Renée Zellweger is the lovable Bridget Jones. To mark the start of the New Year and help to keep her accountable, Bridget starts keeping a diary. The case for perfect imperfection is made exceptionally through this character's witty antics. Despite many work and personal mishaps, Bridget avoids being hard on herself, embracing the fact that as humans we are all flawed. Interestingly, Bridget was the only fictional character that made the BBC Radio 4 Woman's Hour Power List 2016. Bridget's vulnerabilities and humanness are exactly why we connect with this character, and as with all good art, we learn more about our own relationship with perfection. We learn through Bridget that there is no courage without showing vulnerability, and by being authentic, we develop a better relationship with ourselves and others.

Perfectly Imperfect

Brené Brown, a professor at the University of Houston, studies shame, vulnerability, courage, and perfectionism. In her book *The Gifts of Imperfection* (Brown 2010), she breaks down the perils of perfectionism and identifies the key characteristics of authentic, wholehearted living:

- Perfection is a maladaptive protective mechanism where we combat feeling not enough by pleasing, performing, and putting on a mask.
- We can think of it as an armour to protect ourselves and prevent us feeling hurt, but in truth it keeps us from being seen.
- The internal thought process is 'If I look perfect, I can avoid criticism, blame, and ridicule'.

- We struggle in areas of perfectionism where we feel most vulnerable to shame. Shame is the intensely uncomfortable feeling that we are unworthy of love and belonging. It is the most primitive human emotion we all feel.
- Healthy striving is internally focused – being the best I can be – whereas perfectionism is driven by what people will think.
- Authentic wholehearted individuals, according to Brown's research, show qualities of self-compassion and authenticity, lean on others for support, have strong social connections, show gratitude, have the courage to be imperfect, are open to sharing vulnerabilities, show spirituality, practise mindfulness, and set boundaries.

Did You Know?

Kintsugi is the ancient Japanese art of repairing fractured pottery with gold lacquer. It is also a wonderful metaphor for life – we can forge a new relationship with our flaws, learn to love all of our eccentricities, and create a masterpiece celebrating every part, including all the 'cracks'. Looking out for beauty in imperfection is an excellent reframe in counteracting perfectionism.

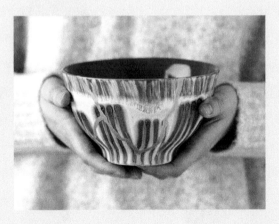

One of the challenges to self-compassion for dental professionals is that patients also expect perfect systems, leaving little room for error. However, without self-compassion and accepting our humanity, we run the risk of flagellating ourselves for every error. In the rest of this chapter, we explore how to use self-compassion to counteract self-perfection and nurture a kinder, softer inner voice.

Delving into the Detail

Three Elements of Self-compassion

Self-compassion practices encourage us to foster an inner ally rather than a bully. The psychologist and key researcher in self compassion Kristin Neff describes three core components of self-compassion: mindfulness, common humanity, and self-kindness (Neff 2003).

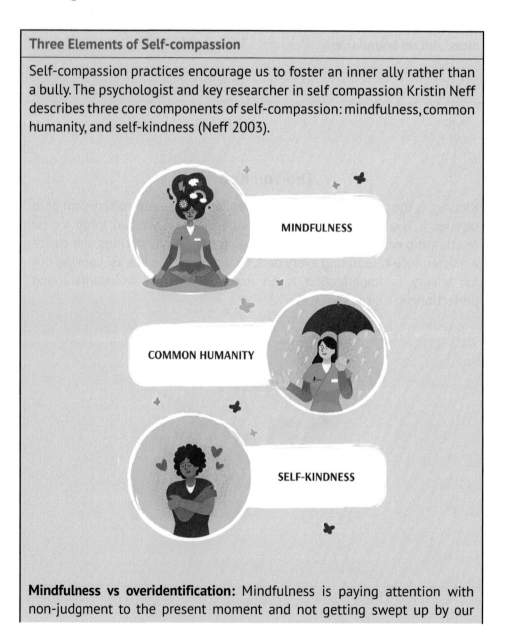

MINDFULNESS

COMMON HUMANITY

SELF-KINDNESS

Mindfulness vs overidentification: Mindfulness is paying attention with non-judgment to the present moment and not getting swept up by our negative thinking traps and emotions nor trying to avoid them. It is the first step to working the self-compassion muscle! When we buy into the story of our thoughts, we are prone to getting swept up by them and believe those thoughts to be true. Being mindful results in us taking the observer role.

Negative emotions are to be expected in life. When we fight our experience and resist our natural emotions, often the pain of those emotions and feelings persists. It becomes resistance. We may note that our attention wanders; we may have physical tension in the body, worry, rumination, defensiveness; or we may seek distraction. We can be happier if we learn to live with less resistance. So, how can mindfulness aid the self-compassion building process?

The mindfulness component of self-compassion allows us to know we are suffering and therefore allows us to lean into self-kindness and have a tender response towards our pain. It is the first step towards self-compassion. Mindfulness also allows us to accept our negative emotions over resisting them.

Common humanity over isolation: Common humanity involves understanding that we all share a sense of interconnectedness, all dental professionals make mistakes and are works in progress, and we all experiences stress.

Self-kindness over self-criticism: This is an approach of offering ourselves warmth and unconditional acceptance when there are challenges. In dentistry, treatments sometimes do not go according to plan and are difficult in complexity, or management of patients can be stressful in nature – for example, managing anxious patients or patients with high expectations. As opposed to using a harsh inner critical voice if things do not go smoothly (a root fractures whilst we are taking a tooth out, we fall short of the working length of an RCT, or we run terribly behind all morning), self-kindness leans towards fostering a soothing and comforting inner voice. We all have skills of self-kindness, often employing it for our friends or children.

Measure Your Well-being: Self-compassion

How do you typically act towards yourself in difficult times? Measure your levels of self-compassion using the self-compassion scale below (adapted from Neff 2003).

Please read each statement carefully before answering. To the left of each item, indicate how often you behave in the stated manner, using the following scale:

Almost never				Almost always
1	2	3	4	5

___1. I'm disapproving and judgmental about my own flaws and inadequacies.

___2. When I'm feeling down I tend to obsess and fixate on everything that's wrong.

___3. When things are going badly for me, I see the difficulties as part of life that everyone goes through.

___4. When I think about my inadequacies, it tends to make me feel more separate and cut off from the rest of the world.

___5. I try to be loving towards myself when I'm feeling emotional pain.

___6. When I fail at something important to me I become consumed by feelings of inadequacy.

___7. When I'm down, I remind myself that there are lots of other people in the world feeling like I am.

___8. When times are really difficult, I tend to be tough on myself.

___9. When something upsets me I try to keep my emotions in balance.

___10. When I feel inadequate in some way, I try to remind myself that feelings of inadequacy are shared by most people.

___11. I'm intolerant and impatient towards those aspects of my personality I don't like.

___12. When I'm going through a very hard time, I give myself the caring and tenderness I need.

___13. When I'm feeling down, I tend to feel like most other people are probably happier than I am.

___14. When something painful happens I try to take a balanced view of the situation.

___15. I try to see my failings as part of the human condition.

___16. When I see aspects of myself that I don't like, I get down on myself.

Measure Your Well-being: Self-compassion

___17. When I fail at something important to me I try to keep things in perspective.

___18. When I'm really struggling, I tend to feel like other people must be having an easier time of it.

___19. I'm kind to myself when I'm experiencing suffering.

___20. When something upsets me I get carried away with my feelings.

___21. I can be a bit cold-hearted towards myself when I'm experiencing suffering.

___22. When I'm feeling down I try to approach my feelings with curiosity and openness.

___23. I'm tolerant of my own flaws and inadequacies.

___24. When something painful happens I tend to blow the incident out of proportion.

___25. When I fail at something that's important to me, I tend to feel alone in my failure.

___26. I try to be understanding and patient towards those aspects of my personality I don't like.

Coding key:

- Self-kindness items: 5, 12, 19, 23, 26
- Self-judgment items: 1, 8, 11, 16, 21
- Common humanity items: 3, 7, 10, 15
- Isolation items: 4, 13, 18, 25
- Mindfulness items: 9, 14, 17, 22
- Overidentified items: 2, 6, 20, 24.

To calculate a total compassion score, take the mean score of each subscale (after reverse scoring negative subscales [self- judgment, isolation, and overidentification, i.e. 1 = 5, 2 = 4, 3 = 3. 4 = 2, 5 = 1]) and compute a total mean. You can also use individual subscale scores or use the total score. As a rough guide, average scores for the self-compassion scale are around 3.0 on the 1–5 Likert scale, a score of 1–2.5 indicates low self-compassion, 2.5–3.5 indicates moderate, and 3.5–5.0 is an indication of high self-compassion (Neff 2003).

Debunking the Myths

Common misconceptions	Reality
Self-compassion is being self-indulgent and selfish. How can I think of myself when I am a dental professional and my role is to look after patients and be professional and perform at my peak at all times?	Research shows that in being more self-compassionate to ourselves, we are more caring and supportive in our relationships at work and home and protect ourselves from poor mental health, such as burnout, compassion fatigue, anxiety, and depression. Practising self-compassion results in compassion satisfaction and better outcomes for our patients.
Self-compassion is too soft and will make me weak and vulnerable.	Self-compassion is a reliable source of inner strength. Research shows that self-compassionate people are more resilient and better able to tackle adversities, such as trauma, chronic pain, or divorce. When we think of complaints handling, the tool of self-compassion in the moment can really benefit dental professionals in coping with negative thoughts, support us with kindness, and allow us to mindfully navigate the challenge with courage and resilience.
Self-compassion is throwing a pity party.	Self-compassion is in fact an antidote to self-pity. Self-compassion allows us to acknowledge that we are not alone in making our mistakes and that making mistakes is intrinsically human. Research shows that self-compassionate people are more likely to engage in perspective-taking instead of focusing on their own distress and less likely to ruminate on how terrible the situation is.
I need to be hard on myself to achieve great things and motivate myself. Self-compassion is fine for some people, but I have high standards and big goals I want to achieve in my life.	Self-criticism is not an effective long-term motivator. Self-criticism undermines self-confidence and leads to fear of failure. Self-compassionate people, on the other hand, still have high standards but do not criticise themselves when obstacles get in the way or mistakes happen.
Self-compassion does not come natural to me and is not the type of person I am – I will not be able to change.	Self-compassion is learnable, and over time, just like any mind skill, it will feel more natural. Since the brain is neuroplastic and self-compassion is a muscle we can train, we can rewire the brain through regular practice. The first step is to recognise how you respond to failure and choose the three elements of self-compassion instead of self-criticism, rather than overidentifying with our thoughts and believing that negative events only happen to us.

Scientific Benefits of Self-compassion

What are the benefits of practising self-compassion for dental professionals? There is evidence to support the numerous benefits of self-compassion on our resilience and psychological well-being. Individuals that are more self-compassionate have greater happiness, life satisfaction, motivation, better relationships, and physical health, in addition to reducing their risk of compassion fatigue and poor mental health (see Table 7.1). Self-compassion training for healthcare professionals specifically has been shown to be effective in reducing stress and anxiety and enhancing positive well-being states.

Table 7.1 Summary of research on transformative effects of self-compassion.

Outcome	Research
Negative well-being states	• High self-compassion leads to fewer negative states, such as depression, anxiety, stress, and shame (Macbeth and Gumley 2012; Neff and Germer 2018; Johnson and O'Brien 2013). • In a mindful self-compassion programme intervention study for healthcare professionals, a reduction of burnout and secondary traumatic stress was reported (Neff et al. 2020).
Positive well-being states	• High self-compassion leads to positive well-being states of happiness, optimism, gratitude, authenticity, and life satisfaction (Breen et al. 2010; Gunnell et al. 2017; Yang et al. 2019; Zhang et al. 2020). • Increase in self-compassion and well-being maintained at three months postintervention of a mindful self-compassion programme for healthcare professionals (Neff et al. 2020).
Risk of compassion fatigue	Reduced risk of compassion fatigue and greater compassion satisfaction in healthcare professionals (therapists, nurses, medics, midwives [Atkinson et al. 2017; Richardson et al. 2016; Trocket et al, 2021]).
Health-related behaviour	Increase engagement in health-related behaviours resulting in better overall physical health and immune function due to increased parasympathetic system and reduced sympathetic nervous system activation (Biber and Ellis 2017; Homan and Sirois 2017).
Resilience	Greater resilience to cope with life's challenges.
Sleep	Less sleep disturbance among healthcare professionals (Kemper et al. 2015).

Table 7.1 (Continued)

Outcome	Research
Relationships	Better relationships (Neff and Beretvas 2013).
Self-confidence	More self-confidence.
Motivation	Greater motivation to improve after failure and take greater responsibility for mistakes (Neff et al. 2005).
Imposter syndrome	Less likely to suffer from imposter syndrome (Patzak et al. 2017).
Ability to learn self-compassion	• Self-compassion can be learned – a study of healthcare professionals found mindfulness training increased participants' self-compassion and reduced stress (Shapiro et al. 2005). • Six weeks of online self-compassion training decreased stress and enhanced emotional regulation and well-being in therapists in training (Finlay-Jones et al. 2017).

How to Practise Self-compassion

The following activities are designed to help you apply the science of self-compassion to working with patients and your team members and at home.

Developing a Kinder Inner Voice

Try the journaling activity below (adapted from Neff and Germer 2018) to develop a more self-compassionate inner voice, no matter what your starting point is currently. For a guided meditation of this activity, try the *Discovering Your Compassionate Voice* meditation available on the companion website.

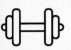

Developing A Kinder Inner Voice

(adapted from Neff and Germer 2018)

1. **Imagine your colleague has come to you distraught and upset.** The colleague has received a patient complaint after completing the first stage of a root canal. The patient is in pain and has called the practice to make a verbal complaint. What types of things would you be saying to your colleague in this situation? What non-verbal responses would you show – for example, physical gestures, tone of voice, how you hold your body?

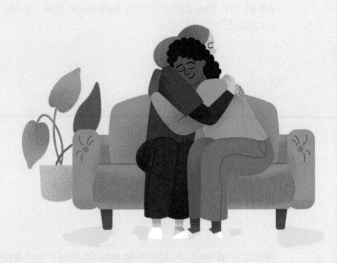

2. **Now imagine if that incident happened to you.** What words would you say to yourself? What non-verbal communication would you show?

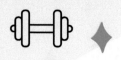

Developing A Kinder Inner Voice

(adapted from Neff and Germer 2018)

3. What are the differences between the words you use with friends and with yourself?

4. What kind and comforting words and non-verbal communication can you offer to yourself instead?

Loving-Kindness Meditation

A Buddhist meditation practice used to specifically build the muscle of self-compassion is Loving-Kindness Meditation (LKM). This self-compassion mindfulness practice, adapted from Buddhist teaching, combines powerful imagery with positive mantras in order to develop feelings of goodwill, kindness, and warmth towards ourselves and others (Salzberg 1995). It uses the power of words, concentration, connection, and caring to do so.

Benefits of LKM

The benefits of LKM include the following:

- Increase feelings of self-compassion, empathy, joy, and gratitude
- Increase levels of positive emotions that outpace the rat race of life
- Increase life satisfaction
- Change our brain regions related to emotional regulation
- Improve our relationships with patients, the dental team, and at home.

LKM can benefit dental professionals in several ways. Firstly, we learn to give ourselves non-judgmental, unconditional kindness. Secondly, we familiarise ourselves with our own pain and suffering, and hence the more we understand the quiet suffering in others. This in turn has enormous 360° benefits, enhancing our relationships with our empathy with patients, the dental team, and at home.

Studies validate that LKM increases our feelings of self-compassion alongside empathy, joy, and gratitude. In one particular study, this increase in positive emotions was noted for up to seven weeks postintervention (Fredrickson et al. 2008). Furthermore, LKM appears to produce positive emotions that outpace the 'rat race' treadmill effect many of us report. It is thought to do so based upon Barbara Fredrickson's Broaden-and-Build Theory, where an increase in positive emotions increases our resources and hence our life satisfaction. LKM also changes our brain structure. Leung et al. (2013) reported an increase in grey matter in areas of the brain related to emotional regulation in Loving-Kindness meditators (right angular posterior parahippocampal gyri).

Soothing Our Bodies Using Self-compassion

Harsh self-criticism activates our sympathetic nervous system and elevates our stress hormones. When we criticise ourselves, we tap into the body's threat mechanism – fight, flight, and freeze. This part of the brain (amygdala) was developed to keep us safe; however, nowadays the threats are not external. The threats are more about our self-concept; for example, as a result of comparing our clinical work with another dental professional on Instagram. Self-compassion, on the other hand, can activate our biologically soothing signals (Gilbert 2005). It allows us to feel connected to others and ourselves through the release of oxytocin and opiates. Soothing and supportive touch evokes ease and well-being. Examples include stroking arms, cupping hands, hugs, hand on heart, and cupping hands on lap or our cheek. Loving and kind inner language, such as words or mantras that are supportive, also does this. Alternatively, we can use self-compassion meditations or self-compassion journaling.

Acts of Self-compassion

We can offer ourselves compassion through leaning towards behaviours that are kinder and supportive to us. Below are some practical examples of how we can take compassionate actions when with patients and at home.

- Resting intentionally – scheduling in regular chunks of downtime rather than a day packed to the brim.
- Paying attention to what brings us joy and doing more of it.
- Celebrating our wins.
- Feeding ourselves with nutritious food.
- Prioritising exercise.
- Taking phone and screen breaks.
- Going to bed early and practising sleep hygiene.
- Taking regular deep breaths at work whilst with patients and practising mindfulness meditation at home.
- Giving ourselves a hug or a soothing squeeze of the arm when we feel stressed during difficult clinical procedures.
- Saying no when we are at full capacity.
- Working on setting boundaries.
- Asking for help and seeking support from family, friends, and mentors.
- Giving ourselves permission to be imperfect.
- When 'failures' arise with dental treatment, reminding ourselves that we can learn great lessons here and keep improving.
- Reframing negative self-talk without judgment and reminding ourselves that with time and effort we can train our brain to become more self-compassionate.
- Forgiving ourselves.

Loving-Kindness Meditation

LOVING-KINDNESS MEDITATION

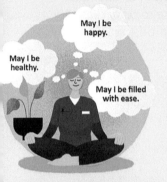

May I be healthy.

May I be happy.

May I be filled with ease.

HOW DOES IT WORK?

- Sit comfortably with your eyes closed. Be ready with the phrases you'll direct to yourself and others.

- Direct kindness and compassion to yourself by repeating a thought like, 'May I be happy'.

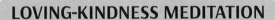

NEXT, DIRECT LOVING KINDNESS TOWARDS...

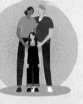
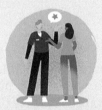
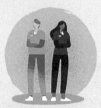

FAMILY AND FRIENDS **SOMEONE NEUTRAL** **SOMEONE DIFFICULT**

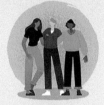
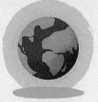

GROUP **EVERYONE**

1. Find a comfortable space to sit down and close your eyes.
2. Take a deep breath in, allowing your mind to settle. Notice the sensation of your breath.
3. Direct loving kindness to yourself, with every breath. You can imagine a warm yellow glow filling your lungs and your entire body.
4. Say to yourself, 'May I be happy, May I be healthy, May I be filled with ease'. Alternatively, use any words that provide comfort and resonate with you the best.
5. Now direct this loving, kind, warm glow towards a loved one. Say to yourself, 'May you be happy, May you be healthy, May you be filled with ease'.
6. Direct your attention to someone neutral, like a work colleague. Repeat, 'May you be happy, May you be healthy, May you be filled with ease'. Keep in mind the warm glow exchange as you direct loving kindness.
7. Direct your attention to someone you find difficult or don't get along with. Repeat, 'May you be happy, May you be healthy, May you be filled with ease'.
8. Finally, direct your attention to the world. Repeat, 'May all beings be happy, May all beings be healthy, May all beings be filled with ease'.

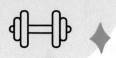

Choosing The Right Words

(adapted from Neff and Germer 2018)

The language we use and the words we adopt to talk to ourselves are really powerful. LKM encourages us to exchange words that hurt us to words of kindness. The mantra used in your LKM needs to feel simple and kind, capture an element of a wish, and, most importantly, be words that speak to you in an authentic and deep way. Try the worksheet below to help you choose the words that resonate with you.

1. **Reflect on what you really need presently and write this down.** For example, to feel like you are a competent dental professional, the desire to be accepted by your colleagues and patients, to feel like you are worthy of this position.

2. **Reflect on what you long to hear from others.** It could be from your work colleagues, friends, or family; for example, I believe you always put your patients' interests first, I trust your clinical judgment, you always take time out to help others, you are so thoughtful in your clinical decisions.

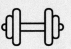

Choosing The Right Words

(adapted from Neff and Germer 2018)

3. **Now frame the above desires as a blessing for yourself.** For example, may I trust my clinical judgment, may I have faith that I keep improving in my clinical skills, may I know my own strengths. Go on a test run and try your LKM with this new set of mantras!

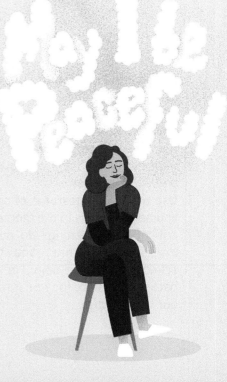

Self-compassion With Patients

Try this three-step process, based on Neff's three pillars of self-compassion, next time you notice stress or anxiety with a patient.

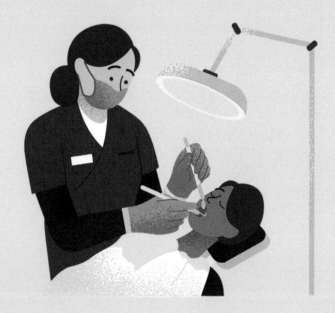

1. **Take a mindful deep breath.** Ensure your exhale is longer than the inhale to trigger your parasympathetic nervous system and invite a sense of calm. Mindfulness prevents us from fusing with our negative thoughts and buying into their story.
2. **Remember that you are not alone in how you are feeling.** This involves understanding that all dental professionals make mistakes, have challenges, and experience stress.
3. **Use words and gestures of self-kindness.** This is an approach of offering yourself kindness in the moment. In dentistry, instead of using a harsh inner critical voice if things do not go smoothly, self-kindness leans towards fostering a soothing and comforting inner voice. We may start by acknowledging the pain: 'I'm so sorry you are experiencing this. I have your back and I'm here for you'. It may involve soothing touch, such as squeezing our hand or arm.

For guided meditations of all of the above activities, see the companion website.

Summary

- Perfectionism traits appear to be high amongst dental professionals and are linked to psychological distress and unhelpful coping strategies.
- Perfectionism is linked with procrastination.
- Self-compassion is an antidote to perfectionism and common negative thoughts.
- Self-compassion means loving kindness directed inwards.
- Three components of self-compassion include mindfulness, common humanity, and self-kindness.
- Self-compassion has numerous well-being benefits: it increases positive well-being states; decreases negative well-being states; reduces risk of compassion fatigue; increases health-related behaviours, sleep, relationships, and self-confidence; and helps to counteract imposter syndrome.
- We can practise self-compassion through meditations, journaling, offering ourselves words of self-kindness, soothing touch, and compassionate actions.
- LKM combines mindfulness with imagery and positive affirmations.
- We can use mindful self-compassion with our patients in the moment of stress by taking a mindful breath, remembering we not alone in how we are feeling, and using words and gestures of self-kindness.

 The View From Here

The final part of the EI discussion saw us delve deep into how self-compassion can help dentistry. Having coached many dental professionals and taught self-compassion in programmes, I am well aware of how this mighty positive emotion has the enormous potential of enhancing patient care and helping us respond to ourselves with the appropriate kindness we infrequently give to ourselves. With its benefits in reducing burnout and compassion fatigue, as well as boosting our compassion satisfaction, happiness levels, motivation, life satisfaction, relationships, and physical health, investing in practising mindful self-compassion really pays off! The number one barrier to self-compassion in dental professionals tends to be individuals believing they need to be self-critical in order to be the best clinician they can be, to stay motivated for upskilling, and to perform the 'perfect' treatment for patients. The research unequivocally shows otherwise: self-compassion is a much more effective motivator long term than the inner critic.

The inner critic, of course, is not the enemy. It is a part of ourselves evolved to keep us safe and in control. Getting to understand the facets of our inner critic, how it shows up in us, and how it thinks it is helping us can with time allow us to label the inner critic and provide some distance between us and the negative thought. The more we relate to it compassionately, the more we can be released from its grip.

Self-compassion is a lifelong journey. It encourages us to ask ourselves, everyday, *How am I treating myself? Am I speaking to myself and acting in a way I would towards a loved one? What climate am I creating in my mind? What do I need to help support myself right now?* It certainly isn't always easy. However, once self-compassion is embraced, it could radically change how we relate to ourselves forever.

References

Brown, B. (2010). *The Gifts of Imperfection*. Hazelden Information & Educational Services.

Gilbert, P. (2005). *Compassion: Conceptualisations, Research and Use in Psychotherapy*. Routledge.

Grzegorek, J.L., Slaney, R.B., Franze, S., and Rice, K.G. (2004). Self-criticism, dependency, self-esteem, and grade point average satisfaction among clusters of perfectionists and non perfectionists. *Journal of Counseling Psychology* 51: 192–200.

Johnson, E. and O'Brien, K. (2013). Self-compassion soothes the savage EGO-threat system: effects on negative affect, shame, rumination, and depressive symptoms. *Journal of Social and Clinical Psychology.* 32 (9): 939–963.

Mehr, K.E. and Adams, A.C. (2016). Self-compassion as a mediator of maladaptive perfectionism and depressive symptoms in college students. *Journal of College Student Psychotherapy* 30: 132–145.

Neff, K.D. (2003). Development and validation of a scale to measure self-compassion. *Self and Identity* 2: 223–250.

Neff, K.D. and Beretvas, S.N. (2013). The role of self-compassion in romantic relationships. *Self and Identity* 12 (1): 78–98.

Neff, K. and Germer, C.K. (2018). *The Mindful Self-Compassion Workbook: A Proven Way to Accept Yourself, Build Inner Strength, and Thrive*. Guilford Press.

Neff, K., Knox, M.C., Long, P., and Gregory, K. (2020). Caring for others without losing yourself: an adaptation of the mindful self-compassion program for healthcare communities. *Journal of Clinical Psychology* 76 (9): 1543–1562.

Shapiro, S., Astin, J., Bishop, S., and Cordova, M. (2005). Mindfulness-based stress reduction for health care professionals: results from a randomized trial. *International Journal of Stress Management* 12: 164–176.

Yang, Y., Guo, Z., Kou, Y., and Liu, B. (2019). Linking self compassion and prosocial behavior in adolescents: the mediating roles of relatedness and trust. *Child Indicators Research* 1–15.

Zhang, J.W., Chen, S., and Tomova Shakur, T.K. (2020). From me to you: self-compassion predicts acceptance of own and others' imperfections. *Personality and Social Psychology Bulletin* 46 (2): 228–242.

Atkinson, D.M., Rodman, J., Thuras, P.D. et al. (2017). Examining burnout, depression, and self-compassion in Veterans Affairs mental health staff. *Journal of Alternative and Complementary Medicine* 23 (7): 551–557.

Biber, D.D. and Ellis, R. (2017). The effect of self-compassion on the self-regulation of health behaviors: a systematic review. *Journal of Health Psychology* 24 (14): 2060–2071.

Breen, W.E., Kashdan, T.B., Lenser, M.L., and Fincham, F.D. (2010). Gratitude and forgiveness: convergence and divergence on self-reports and informant ratings. *Personality and Individual Differences* 49: 932–937.

Collin, V., O'Selmo, E., and Whitehead, P. (2020). Stress, psychological distress, burnout and perfectionism in UK dental students. *British Dental Journal* 229 (9): 605–614.

Finlay-Jones, A., Kane, R., and Rees, C. (2017). Self-compassion online: a pilot study of an internet-based self-compassion cultivation program for psychology trainees. *Journal of Clinical Psychology* 73 (7): 797–816.

Fredrickson, B.L., Cohn, M.A., Coffey, K.A. et al. (2008). Open hearts build lives: positive emotions, induced through loving-kindness meditation, build consequential personal resources. *Journal of Personality and Social Psychology* 95 (5): 1045–1062.

Gunnell, K.E., Mosewich, A.D., McEwen, C.E. et al. (2017). Don't be so hard on yourself! Changes in self-compassion during the first year of university are associated with changes in well-being. *Personality and Individual Differences* 107: 43–48.

Hewitt, P.L. and Flett, G.L. (1989). The Multidimensional Perfectionism Scale: development and validation. *Canadian Psychology* 30: 339.

Homan, K.J. and Sirois, F.M. (2017). Self-compassion and physical health: exploring the roles of perceived stress and health-promoting behaviors. *Health Psychology Open* 4 (2).

Kemper, K.J., Mo, X., and Khayat, R. (2015). Are mindfulness and self-compassion associated with sleep and resilience in health professionals? *Journal of Alternative and Complementary Medicine* 21 (8): 496–503.

Leung, M.K., Chan, C.C., Yin, J. et al. (2013). Increased gray matter volume in the right angular and posterior parahippocampal gyri in loving-kindness meditators. *Social Cognitive and Affective Neuroscience* 8 (1): 34–39.

MacBeth, A. and Gumley, A. (2012). Exploring compassion: a meta-analysis of the association between self-compassion and psychopathology. *Clinical Psychology Review* 32 (6): 545–552.

Neff, K.D., Hsieh, Y.-P., and Dejitterat, K. (2005). Self-compassion, achievement goals, and coping with academic failure. *Self and Identity* 4 (3): 263–287.

Patzak, A., Kollmayer, M., and Schober, B. (2017). Buffering impostor feelings with kindness: the mediating role of self-compassion between gender-role orientation and the impostor phenomenon. *Frontiers in Psychology* 8: 1289.

Richardson, D.A., Jaber, S., Chan, S. et al. (2016). Self-compassion and empathy: impact on burnout and secondary traumatic stress in medical training. *Open Journal of Epidemiology* 6: 161–166.

Salzberg, S. (1995). *Loving-Kindness: The Revolutionary Art of Happiness*. Boston, MA: Shambhala.

Trockel, M., Sinsky, C., West, C.P. et al. (2021). Self-valuation challenges in the culture and practice of medicine and physician well-being. *Mayo Clinic Proceedings* 96 (8): 2123–2132.

8

Resilient Mindset

CHAPTER OVERVIEW

- Importance of resilient thinking styles in dentistry
- Identifying our thinking traps
- Using cognitive behavioural therapy as a dental professional
- Developing an optimistic mindset
- Compassionate mindset
- Growth mindset.

Each one of us is like that butterfly, the Butterfly Effect. And each tiny move toward a more positive mindset can send ripples of positivity through our organisations, our families and our communities.

—Shawn Achor, author of *The Happiness Advantage*

Mindset refers to a pattern of thinking and beliefs we hold about ourselves. These thinking patterns are hugely influential in determining our emotions, our behaviours, and our perception of the world. Developing a resilient mindset for dental professionals means fostering thinking patterns that allow us to adapt and weather stress or challenges at work. This type of mindset also allows us to grow through obstacles and thrive. In this chapter, we delve into the 'R' of the PERLE Resilience Model, spotlighting how dental professionals can apply the interesting insights from the psychology of mindset to work. Specifically, I refer to three types of mindset that are beneficial for dental professionals: optimistic, compassionate, and growth.

A useful way of thinking about mindsets is that our thought patterns lie somewhere along a continuum – with one end representing optimistic, compassionate, and growth orientated, and the other end pessimistic, critical, and fixed. We may be critical in certain areas of our lives but more growth orientated in others. The good news is, no matter where we lie on the continuum, we can shift towards positive mindsets that boost positive emotions and positive actions.

Resilience and Well-being for Dental Professionals, First Edition. Mahrukh Khwaja.
© 2023 John Wiley & Sons Ltd. Published 2023 by John Wiley & Sons Ltd.
Companion website: www.wiley.com/go/khwaja-resilience-dentistry

Before we can delve into nurturing these three mindsets in dentistry, we start with exploring the psychology of thinking and recognising our own thinking traps.

The Board of Directors That Lives in Our Head

A common misunderstanding around our thoughts is our belief that they are accurate. In fact, our brain generates automatic negative thoughts (ANTs) whenever any event happens. This includes mental images that are spontaneous, fleeting, often feel unquestionable, and reflect core beliefs we formed as a child. I like to think of ANTs as a board of directors that lives in our head. Not always useful but trying to take control of the situation. ANTs were evolved to keep us safe from predators. However, in today's modern world, these 'directors' are more like thinking traps that can hijack our brains. Increasing our awareness of which thinking trap we fall into is the first step to nurturing resilient thinking.

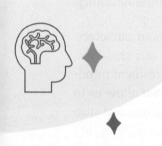

Think About It

What common negative thoughts do you have around work? Do any of these sound familiar?

- I should be perfect at this by now.
- I am going to fail like I usually do.
- That RCT was a disaster. I'm going to get a complaint.
- There's no point in trying.
- That crown prep looked terrible. The crown will never fit.
- Everyone is so much better than me at this.
- Everyone is so much faster than me.

Types of Thinking Traps

Thinking traps, otherwise known as cognitive distortions, are unhelpful patterns of thinking that are often inaccurate and negatively biased. Researchers have identified many thinking traps. The most common thinking traps for dental professionals are summarised in Figure 8.1. Do any of the thinking traps resonate? When I coach dental professionals, I notice that catastrophising is the most common thinking trap, including the 'me' trap.

Common thinking traps for dental professionals

Them trap (blaming) - The converse of the 'me' trap. We believe that the sole cause of the problem is others, completely discounting internal factors.

Catastrophising - Excessive worrying (ruminating) around the worst-case scenario of a situation. This runaway train of thoughts predicts that the negative event will be catastrophic. Catastrophising is closely correlated with anxiety.

Mind telepathy - Jumping to conclusions and assuming we know what the other person is thinking, often negatively, or expecting others to know what we are thinking. This thinking trap has big consequences when it comes to our interpersonal relationships.

Me trap (personalisation) - We believe that the sole cause of the problem is because of our failures. We completely discount any external factors.

Helplessness - We avoid trying because we believe we are doomed to failure. Thoughts such as 'I can't do it, why bother?', that will never work, what's the point?' are examples.

Labelling – Assigning negative labels to ourselves or others, e.g. 'I'm not smart'.

Disqualifying the positive – Discounting the good moments, e.g. saying to yourself, 'that doesn't count'.

Figure 8.1   Common thinking traps.

Understanding Our Triggers

Self-awareness of our triggers for specific thinking traps is essential in regulating our emotions. A common trigger in dentistry may be receiving an unclear message from your work colleagues, such as your receptionist leaving a message to say that a patient wants you to call back, without giving further details. This scenario is one that could quite quickly trigger a runaway catastrophic spiral of thoughts, leading to a General Dental Council (GDC) complaint, all in the space of a few anxious seconds. Other triggers for stress include situations we fear, such as when we are in the middle of complex treatments with our patients, when we are managing a difficult patient, when something we value highly is at stake, or when we are exhausted.

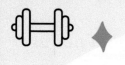

Identify Thinking Traps

1. Think of a time where you felt stressed at work over the last month. Write down what your thoughts were below.

2. Look back at the thinking traps in Figure 8.1. Are any of your thoughts representative of the common thinking traps? What patterns do you observe?

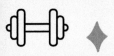

Identify Thinking Traps

3. What was the consequence of thinking this way? Did it prevent you from taking certain actions, or which emotions did it lead to?

Cognitive-Behavioural Therapy

Contrary to popular belief, CBT can be used for both mental illness and to enhance resilience and well-being. CBT is not only for those who are unwell. The thinking-behavioural model (cognitive behavioural therapy; see Figure 8.2) has a special place in psychology in highlighting an important relationship: our thoughts, feelings, and actions. Underpinning these three strands are our deep-rooted underlying core beliefs about ourselves, the world, and other people. As a child, our core beliefs helped us navigate the world and are translated into behaviour or coping strategies. They fall under three categories: helplessness, lovability, and worth. Although they helped us in the past, our fallback strategies may not be so useful as an adult.

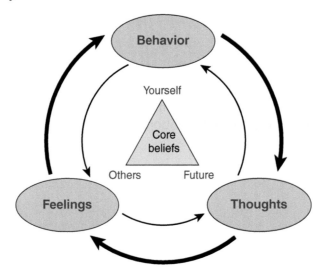

Figure 8.2   CBT model. Adapted from Beck 1964 and Ellis 1957.

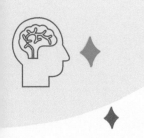

Think About It

Have you noticed the interplay between your beliefs, thoughts, and emotions with your own actions? Sometimes a negative event can trigger a number of negative thoughts that can lead to us to feel anxious, fearful, or angry. This may result in unhelpful behaviours, such as withdrawal, lashing out, or overeating.

There is an enormous amount of evidence to support the CBT model. This research shows that although changing our behaviours is one mighty task, we can influence our thoughts. This can indirectly impact our emotions and thereby our actions. When we think about adversities, having the tool to be flexible with our thinking is very useful. Resilient thinking can buffer us from getting stuck in negative thoughts and help us to shift our attention to thoughts that will help us thrive.

Applying Your ABCs

Understanding how our thoughts and emotions influence how we act can be a very powerful way of preventing being messed around by the events in our life. One way we can do this is using the ABCDE approach (Ellis 1962, 1976; Seligman 1991).

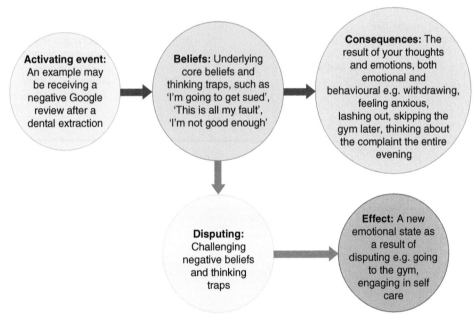

Here are ways we can dispute our unhelpful thoughts:

- **Examining the evidence:** Take your thoughts to court! Reflect on the evidence for and against this thought. How accurate is this thought? Start fleshing out your response using the sentence, 'That's not true because. . .' Really pad this out with real concrete examples that counteract the accuracy of the negative thought.
- **Reframing the unhelpful thought:** This involves thinking of ways of thinking about the scenario in a more positive, helpful way. You can use the statement, 'A more helpful way of thinking about this is. . .' to help you challenge a negative perspective.
- **Planning a backup:** Think about a backup plan if that thought does indeed come true using the sentence, 'If this happens I will. . .'

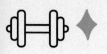

Dispute Unhelpful Thoughts

1. Following on from the previous example in *Identify Thinking Traps*, what ways can you dispute the thinking traps you identified? Note ways you can reframe the thought by thinking of a more helpful way of looking at things, examining the evidence against this thought, and thinking of the best-case scenario.

Negative thought	That's not true because...	A more helpful way to look at this...	The best-case scenario is...
I won't ever be able to do this procedure	*I felt the same way about molar RCTs and now I feel confident with them*	*With time and effort, I can get better*	*I will book onto a course and with practice and support, I will become proficient and enjoy the challenge*

Dispute Unhelpful Thoughts

2. What consequence would this lead to, having challenged those thoughts? Think about the emotional impact as well as the impact on your actions.

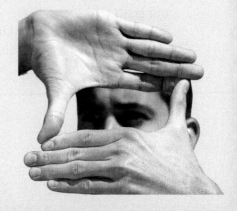

Catch It, Check It, and Change It

There are moments when we may feel emotionally triggered when we are with patients. Having a practical set of thinking tools to use in the moment can be life changing. We can think of this as resilience in real time. Real-time resilience is a concept described by Karen Reivich and Andrew Shatté, in which we apply resilient thinking in the moment, whilst we are feeling stressed or triggered emotionally (Reivich and Shatté 2002). We can apply this by using three steps, the 3Cs: Catch it, Check it, and Change it.

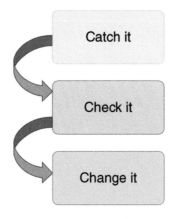

1) **Catch it:** We can catch our thoughts through noticing and labelling them. We may say to ourselves: "I notice I'm having a thought that. . ."
2) **Check it:** Consider whether the thought is helping or hindering you.
3) **Change it:** This refers to disputing the unhelpful thought using the techniques we discussed in the precious section, for example, looking at the evidence, reframing, or planning.

This is a CBT tool we can use in real time, such as when we are with our patients. The impact of this thinking tool is vast. We may feel more optimistic and less anxious, and our well-being and resilience are enhanced. If we think differently, we feel differently too, and this in turn means we act differently. Great news if our mission is to feel good, build our resilience, and pursue our goals.

Another aspect to thinking more resiliently is developing an optimistic mindset. In the next section, we explore what the science says about the benefits of optimism.

Optimistic Mindset

We all encounter challenges, big or small, during our lifetimes. Optimism is the juice that keeps us going. Defined as a set of thoughts that shape how we feel about a positive, hopeful future, optimism has a number of wide-ranging benefits. An optimistic mindset is far from being unrealistic and discounting reality; it is more about inviting more positivity through modifying the lens we see things through.

Glass Half Full or Half Empty?

How do you respond to a crushing blow? How do you handle stress of everyday life? Optimists' thinking skills – that is, identifying problems, viewing situations as challenges and not threats, and identifying what they can control – makes them more capable of managing life's setbacks. Optimists tend to step in and seek solutions, look for information that can help them, and welcome support. Regarding behaviours, optimists take action and are more likely to eat healthily and exercise regularly.

Measure Your Well-being
Optimism

How optimistic are you? Measure your optimism levels using the Life Orientation Test (adapted from Scheier et al. 1994).

For each statement, indicate the response that best applies to you using the following scale.

I disagree a lot		Neutral		I agree a lot
0	1	2	3	4

___1. In uncertain times, I usually expect the best.
___2. It's easy for me to relax.
___3. If something can go wrong for me, it will. (R)
___4. I'm always optimistic about my future.
___5. I enjoy my friends a lot.
___6. It's important for me to keep busy.
___7. I hardly ever expect things to go my way. (R)
___8. I don't get upset too easily.
___9. I rarely count on good things happening to me. (R)
___10. Overall, I expect more good things to happen to me than bad.

Scoring:
Items 3, 7, and 9 are reverse scored. Reversing a score is done by exchanging the original value of an item by its opposite value; for example, a score of 1 turns into a score of 5, a score of 2 turns into a 4, and so forth. Items 2, 5, 6, and 8 are fillers and should not be scored. Add the scores to get your final optimism level.

Score range:
0–13 = Low optimism (high pessimism)
14–18 = Moderate optimism
19–24 = High optimism (low pessimism)

Three Ps of Optimism

Three thinking patterns characterise optimism. When 'good' or 'bad' events happen to us, our brains try to work out why. Our brain may try to work out the cause for the event, and whether it occurred solely because of something wrong we did or to external factors. This is known as personalisation. An optimistic person will consider that the event is not entirely due to them, and that other external factors are in play. Secondly, the brain may also focus on how long lasting the negative effects will be, known as permanence. Optimists realise that bad situations are temporary. Thirdly, our brain focuses on how much the event will impact our life – will it affect one aspect or all parts of our life – known as pervasiveness. Optimists believe that a negative event will impact part of our life but not every aspect. These 3 Ps of optimism make up the explanatory style theory (Seligman 1991).

	Good event	Bad event
Optimist	Permanent	Temporary
	Pervasive	Specific
	Personal (internal)	External cause
Pessimist	Temporary	Permanent
	Specific	Pervasive
	External cause	Personal (internal)

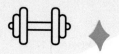

Optimism In Action

One way to apply optimism in a practical way is to think about areas in your life that you can and cannot control. Optimists are very good at identifying control areas, and this helps them feel more hopeful about a positive future, through taking action.

1. Think of a situation you are struggling with currently. Write aspects of the situation you can control and aspects you have no influence on.

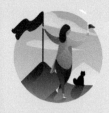

2. Finally, list purposeful actions as small steps that you can take to make the situation better.

Small steps I can take	Alternative steps I can take to help me achieve my goal if challenges arise
✦	
✦	
✦	✦
	✦
✦	✦
✦	✦

Compassionate Mindset

We can be our own worst critics at times. A compassionate mindset is a set of thinking patterns, skills, and attributes that allow dental professionals to invite kindness and warmth, strength, and courage towards ourselves over self-criticism. We can practise self-compassion through meditations, journaling, offering ourself words of self-kindness, and soothing touch. To learn how we can develop this mindset in detail, see Chapter 7.

Growth Mindset

To develop positive habits, to build resilience and well-being, we need to adopt a mindset that can embrace hurdles, prop us up when we are failing, and help us keep learning new skills in dentistry. As discussed in the chapter on self-compassion (Chapter 7), many dental professionals have perfectionistic traits and a harsh inner critic. This can lead us to have a fixed mindset: one where we believe our intelligence is fixed, we focus on mistakes as proof of incompetence, and we even avoid challenges to prevent damage to our sense of self. The alternative type of mindset, known as growth mindset, is a type of positive self-talk where individuals believe that their intelligence and talent are dynamic and ever improving. This mindset can help us unlock a kinder, supportive voice whilst we are upskilling and maintaining our clinical expertise. Without a growth mindset approach, sitting with the discomfort of learning something new, from short-term orthodontics and bonding to occlusion and managing difficult restorative cases, is just not possible.

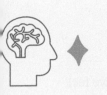

Think About It

Our Inner Voice

Have you ever thought about the type of inner voice you have? Is it critical when you make mistakes? Do you notice it being harsh when you approach a challenge? Does the voice encourage you to give up when the going gets tough?

The inner voice and mindset have been studied with great curiosity, especially by American professor Carol Dweck. Growth mindset was born from studying school children (Dweck 1999). Dweck noted that some of her students in her studies approached challenges with excitement and sense of opportunity. These students possessed a growth mindset, a set of thoughts that acknowledged and embraced their weaknesses, reframed criticism as feedback, and prioritised learning above seeking approval. Success of others felt inspiring. They understood failure distinctly as an opportunity to grow. Students with a growth mindset persisted despite challenges. Students, however, who approached things from a fixed mindset believed that their knowledge was static. They understood failure as a limit of their own ability. This meant that these students often gave up easily.

GROWTH MINDSET

Is Freedom

Persevere in the face of failures
Effort is required to build new skills
Find inspiration in others' success
Embrace challenges
Accept criticism
Desire to learn
Build abilities

FIXED MINDSET

Is Limiting

Avoid challenges
Give up easily
Threatened by others' success
Desire to look smart
Effort is fruitless
Ignore feedback
Fixed abilities

Fixed versus Growth Mindset

As we discussed earlier on in this chapter, what we think impacts how we feel and our actions. Growth mindset thoughts actually make us think, feel, and act very differently.

Impact of Growth Mindset on How We Think, Feel, and Act

Think	Feel	Act
This challenge is an opportunity to learn.	I feel curious and excited by the prospect of new challenges.	I persist during obstacles and do not give up easily.
Failure is an opportunity to grow.	When I stumble, I do not feel like I'm not good enough.	I give and receive constructive criticism.
If they can do it, so can I.	I feel inspired by the success of others.	I look for support from mentors.
Learning is brain training.	I am energised by learning new things.	I look for new things to learn. I go on courses and conferences and read about the latest developments.
With time and effort, I get better.	I am happy as I reflect on my progress.	I regularly review my progress.
Although I'm not there *yet*, I will be.	The journey feels full of opportunity, surprise, and optimism.	I create a vison board to plan the future and journal about my best possible future.
If I work hard and persist, I will get there.		I focus on my goals – breaking them down into smaller steps.
Feedback helps me grow and get better.	I enjoy hearing constructive feedback and feel excited at the prospect of getting more proficient.	I ask for feedback from peers and mentors. I get support from mentors and teachers.
Getting better takes time, patience, and persistence.		
Failing does not mean I'm good enough. I need to 'fail' to learn, and it is part of the journey.		When I fail, I do not flagellate myself for it. I use mindful self-compassion practices to soothe myself.

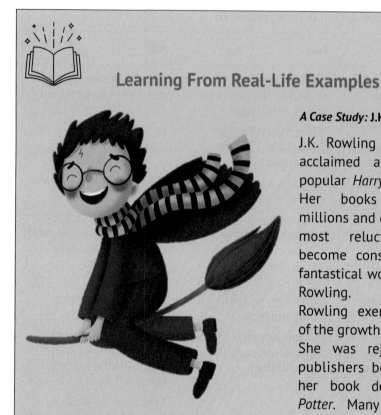

Learning From Real-Life Examples

A Case Study: J.K. Rowling

J.K. Rowling is the world-acclaimed author of the popular *Harry Potter* series. Her books have sold millions and even made the most reluctant readers become consumed by the fantastical world created by Rowling. Interestingly, Rowling exemplifies many of the growth mindset traits. She was rejected by 12 publishers before she got her book deal for *Harry Potter*. Many would have given up after such a large number of rejections, but Rowling believed that although she wasn't there *yet,* she would be. It was this persistence to keep going despite setbacks, to use feedback as a positive, and to believe that hard work and persistence would help her achieve her goals – a true growth mindset attitude – that helped Rowling become arguably one of the most recognised and celebrated authors of today.

Nurturing a Growth Mindset

Dweck discovered that growth mindset was teachable. Drawing from the research on neuroplasticity, once she taught students that they all had the capacity to change their brains through mind training, students felt able to lean towards a growth mindset approach. We can all lean towards a growth mindset through several strategies. These are described below.

1) **Positive language:** The words we use for our inner voice determine how we feel and how we behave. To nurture a positive inner voice, start with recognising fixed mindset inner dialogue. This could be through a mindful check-in, asking ourselves what we are thinking and feeling currently.

Alternatively, we may journal our thoughts. Through check-ins and journaling practices, we can start recognising our internal fixed mindset statements, such as 'if I fail, I'm not good enough' or 'if I avoid challenges, others will not doubt me'. We can then acknowledge that mindset is a choice and one that we can control with practice. Lastly, we can practice a growth mindset approach using positive language, such as replacing the word 'failing' with 'learning' and instead of focusing on results, paying attention to effort. When we catch ourselves frustrated that we aren't 'good enough', we can remind ourselves that we are not there *yet*, and its only a matter of time

2) **Reframing:** This thinking technique can help us lean towards a positive perspective. We can say to ourselves, 'A more helpful way to think about this is. . .'

3) **Reading the latest neuroplasticity research:** This reminds us that our brain has the capacity to structurally change with our efforts at any age.

4) **Using positive growth affirmations:** These are short, positive statements or mantras that embody growth mindset; for example, 'mistakes are progress', 'embrace the challenge', and 'learning requires effort'. Positive affirmations have been shown to boost our happiness levels as well as our well-being (Bolier et al. 2013; Sin and Lyubomirsky 2009). We can use these statements during challenging dental treatments, such as a difficult extraction or RCT. They help us shift from a fixed mindset to a growth mindset.

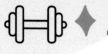

Thrive Using Growth Mindset

1. Reflect on your main triggers for stress during dental treatment.

2. Consider what your current self-talk during dental treatment is. What words do you say to yourself? Are there any patterns? How does it make you think, feel, and act?

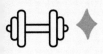

Thrive Using Growth Mindset

3. What are alternative statements you can say, inspired by growth mindset affirmations? Examples include 'When I fail, I learn', 'This might take time and effort', 'I'm not there yet but I will be', 'I strive for progress not perfection', and 'I grow through challenging myself'.

Instead of	Try
If I can't do this, I'll be a failure	*I might not be able to do this the first time, but it's just going to take practise*

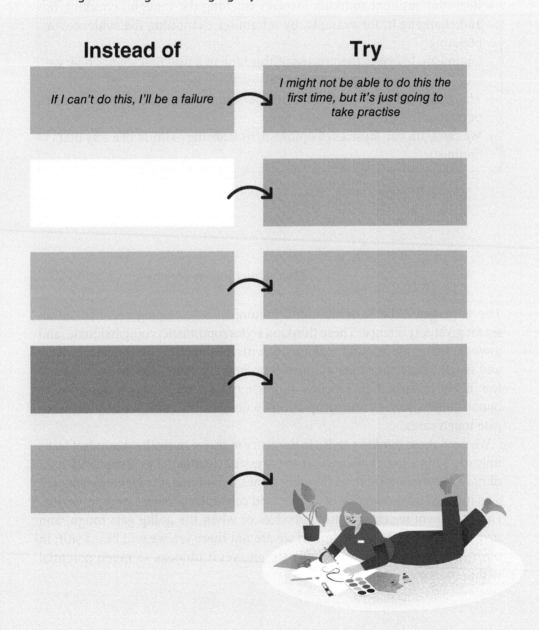

Summary

- We can train our minds to become more resilient.
- The common thinking traps for dental professionals include mind telepathy, me trap, disqualifying the positive helplessness, labelling, them trap, and catastrophising.
- We can counteract these thinking traps using CBT.
- Real-time resilient thinking involves catching the thought, checking it, and changing it, for example, by reframing, examining the evidence, or planning.
- Optimism describes the process of thinking in a way that shapes how we feel about a positive, hopeful future.
- The three pillars of optimism are personalisation, pervasiveness, and permanence.
- We can train our muscles of optimism by learning to think in a way that is optimistic.

 The View From Here

The 'R' of the PERLE Resilience Model illuminates developing a resilient mindset for greater resilience. These thinking styles (optimistic, compassionate, and growth) are highly relevant to dentistry with the opposite (pessimistic, critical, and fixed) having detrimental impacts on how we think, feel and act. We are less likely to upskill as a dental professional otherwise, open ourselves to opportunities, such as setting up our own dental clinic, and successfully navigate tough cases.

We need these thinking styles in dentistry to thrive. A resilient mindset leans towards embracing challenges, from stressful treatments to complaints handling, and reframes them as stepping stones in building greater competencies; gets inspired by the success of others; and celebrates progress over perfection. One statement we can remind ourselves of when the going gets tough, and invariably it will, is that although we are not there *yet*, we will be – a shift in our inner language so deceptively simple, yet it unlocks so much potential within us.

- Optimists see bad events as temporary and specific and attribute external causes.
- We can practise self-compassion through meditations, journaling, offering words of self-kindness, and soothing touch.
- We can adopt a growth mindset through using positive language, reframing, reading neuroplastic research, and using growth affirmations whilst we are upskilling or performing a difficult or new clinical procedure.

References

Beck, J.S. (1964). *Cognitive Therapy: Basics and Beyond*. New York: Guildford Press.

Bolier, L., Haverman, M., Westerhof, G.J. et al. (2013). Positive psychology interventions: a meta-analysis of randomized controlled studies. *BMC Public Health* 13: 119.

Dweck, C.S. (1999). *Mindset: The New Psychology of Success*. New York: Random House.

Ellis, A. (1957). Rational psychotherapy and individual psychology. *Journal of Individual Psychology* 13: 38–44.

Ellis, A. (1962). *Reason and Emotion in Psychotherapy*. Lyle Stuart.

Ellis, A. (1976). RET abolishes most of the human ego. *Psychotherapy* 13: 343–348.

Reivich, K. and Shatté, A. (2002). *The Resilience Factor: 7 Essential Skills for Overcoming Life's Inevitable Obstacles*. Broadway Books.

Scheier, M.F., Carver, C.S., and Bridges, M.W. (1994). Distinguishing optimism from neuroticism (and trait anxiety, self-mastery, and self-esteem): a re-evaluation of the life orientation test. *Journal of Personality and Social Psychology* 67: 1063–1078.

Seligman, M.E.P. (1991). *Learned Optimism: How to Change Your Mind and Your Life*. New York: Pocket Books.

Sin, N.L. and Lyubomirsky, S. (2009). Enhancing well-being and alleviating depressive symptoms with positive psychology interventions: a practice-friendly meta-analysis. *Journal of Clinical Psychology* 65: 467–487.

9

Lifestyle

<table>
<tr><td>

CHAPTER OVERVIEW

- Importance of lifestyle factors in building resilience
- Gut health and well-being
- Mindful eating
- Mindful movement
- Sleep hygiene
- Lessons from Blue Zones.

</td></tr>
</table>

The mind and body are not separate. What affects one, affects the other.

—Anonymous

Positive health can be characterised not only as a long and disease-free life but also less frequent ailments, ability to recuperate, and more physiological reserves. From the growing research, we know that positive psychology characteristics, such as experiencing positive emotions, high levels of optimism, emotional regulation, having a life purpose, positive social relationships, and spirituality, promote positive health and longevity. To integrate positive lifestyle behaviours for the long-term requires a lifestyle change.

As we spotlight in Chapter 1, our mental health protective factors that encourage positive outcomes include lifestyle factors of good nutrition, adequate physical exercise, good-quality sleep, and the avoidance of drugs and smoking. And in this chapter, the 'L' of the PERLE Resilience Model, our lifestyle, is the focus. We start by exploring how, as dental professionals, we can integrate the key findings from lifestyle medicine to build greater resilience.

Nourish by Eating Well

Food is a fuel not just for the body, but also the mind. There is growing evidence that nutrition has links to well-being and optimal functioning. Greater levels of well-being were reported in individuals who ate a diet rich in fruits and vegetables (Rees et al. 2019). The food we eat impacts how we think and behave. See Table 9.1 for mood-boosting vitamins and minerals that can help our physical well-being as well as our psychological wellness.

Table 9.1   Mood-boosting vitamins and minerals.

Vitamin/ mineral	Food	Benefits on mood
Vitamin C	Oranges, kiwi fruit, tomatoes, sweet potato, broccoli, peppers	A well-known antioxidant that is involved in anxiety, stress, depression, fatigue, and mood state in humans. Vitamin C converts tryptophan, an amino acid present in the animal proteins in the diet, into serotonin, a hormone responsible for regulating mood.
Vitamin D	Oily fish, red meat, egg yolks	May play an important role in emotional regulation and warding off depression. In one Norwegian study, researchers reported that participants with depression who received vitamin D supplements improved in their symptoms (Jorde et al. 2008).
Vitamin B12	Meat, milk, cheese, salmon, cod, eggs	Plays a vital role in synthesising and metabolising serotonin.
Iron	Red meat, lentils, dark leafy vegetables	Low levels of iron cause less oxygen to get to our cells, keeping them from functioning properly and often leading to lethargy, weakness, anxiety, and depression.
Folic acid	Green vegetables, oranges and citrus fruits, beans	Helps the body create new cells and supports serotonin regulation.
Omega 3	Oily fish, such as mackerel and salmon	Emerging as effective for mood disorders ranging from major depression and postpartum depression to bipolar disorder and schizophrenia.
Selenium	Brazil nuts, fish, meat, eggs	Elevates mood and decreases anxiety by raising neurotransmitter levels.
Zinc	Meat, milk, shellfish, bread, cheese	Involved in synthetising serotonin and dopamine.

Gut Health and Well-Being

Did you know that keeping your gut healthy may aid in keeping your brain healthy as well? Recently medical literature is increasingly shining a light on the important relationship between our brain and a gut microbiome (microorganisms). Eating poorly may affect the brain through causing symptoms that are similar to anxiety (Messaoudi et al. 2011a, 2011b; Hilimire et al. 2015), depression (Akkasheh et al., 2016), autism, and Parkinson's disease. It does this through preventing us from getting key nutrients to keep healthy. Additionally, a poor diet may damage the composition of the gut microbiome and cause an inability to properly break down nutrients. Stress also greatly contributes here – and the more stressed we are, the more damage we may cause to the gut microbiome. Contrastingly, eating well contributes to creating a healthy gut, full of diverse gut microbiome. We are more likely to get sick less often, be more productive, and have greater emotional well-being.

As with all our body systems, a combination of a diet rich in gut-friendly foods, stress management – for example, regular mindfulness practice and physical exercise – as well as targeted supplements may all aid in creating a gut and brain that are healthy. With regards to positive nutrition, consider increasing the gut-healthy foods in Figure 9.1 on a regular basis.

Mindful Eating

Mindful eating is a type of informal mindfulness practice that we can easily incorporate into our working days. Mindless eating involves eating and multi-tasking or eating past full and ignoring our body's signals. Mindful eating, however, encourages us to slow down to notice the experience of eating.

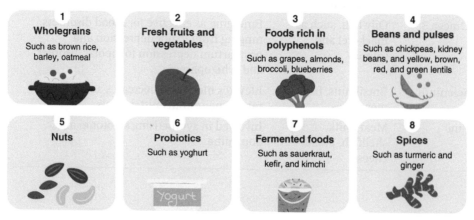

Figure 9.1 Gut-healthy foods.

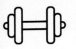

Mindful Eating Challenge

Try this 7-day challenge to practise mindful eating this week. Through this activity, you will exercise your mind muscles of self-compassion, focus, gratitude, and curiosity.

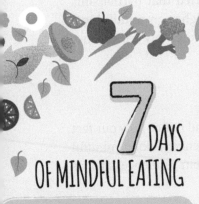

7 DAYS OF MINDFUL EATING

Day 1
JOT DOWN YOUR PLAN
At the start of your week, jot down a quick food plan! While you're shopping or picking up food this week, try to keep your plan in mind!

Day 2
PAUSE AND REFLECT
Halfway through your meal, take a break to check in with your body (this isn't easy!). From 1-10, how full do you feel?

Day 3
HAVE A SEAT
Have a seat. When you can, sit down to eat your food without multi-tasking, even if it's just a snack.

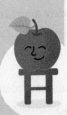

Day 4
HANDY REMINDERS
Consider tying a string around your wrist or wearing a certain bracelet or ring as a gentle reminder to eat mindfully.

Day 5
ENGAGE YOUR SENSES
The next time you're eating, take your first bite with your eyes closed. Notice the texture, the sound of the crunch, and every delicious smell and flavor.

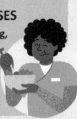

Day 6
BE KIND TO YOURSELF
If you don't have time or energy to approach a meal mindfully, that's OK. Be forgiving with yourself.

Day 7
KEEP PRACTICING
Like meditation, mindful eating is a skill that takes consistent practice. Keep going!

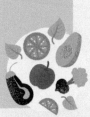

Day 1: Write down a food plan for the week. When you are picking up the shopping, try to keep this plan in mind.

Day 2: Midpoint through your meal, take a moment to pause and check in with your body. From 1–10, how full do you feel?

Day 3: Sit down to eat without your phone or multitasking.

Day 4: Engage all of your senses by noticing the texture, sound, taste, smell, and flavour of your first three bites of food.

Day 5: Use reminders to help you to remember to eat mindfully, such as a mindfulness bell or a bracelet.

Day 6: Be compassionate. If you don't have energy to approach a meal mindfully, that's okay.

Day 7: Keep going! Mindful eating, just like mindfulness meditation, takes practice.

Replenish with Exercise

Increasing movement has been long linked to psychological well-being, with research highlighting decreases in symptoms of anxiety, depression, and loneliness with physical exercise (Hyde et al. 2013). Despite the many reported benefits, it can be difficult as a busy dental professional to integrate more movement in our daily lives.

Mindfulness can be used in exercise to encourage taking up physical exercise and maintaining a positive lifestyle habit. Researchers Ulmer et al. (2010) examined the use of mindfulness in exercise and reported that participants who maintained a longer duration of exercise scored higher on mindfulness and acceptance measures. In the next sections, we explore how we can use mindfulness principles to boost our levels of movement.

Mindful Walking

We can practise mindful walking, where we slow down and notice how our feet feel against the ground and our surroundings with presence. Taking mindful walks encourages a range of positive emotions that boost our resilience, such as awe, curiosity, zest, and self-compassion.

- **Start by bringing your awareness to your body:** Notice how each muscle is involved as you walk. Note how your arms and legs feel as you walk and the sensation of the ground as you move forward and lay each foot down.
- **Bring your awareness to your breath:** Notice your breath as you inhale and exhale, feeling your ribs expand and slowly deflate.
- **Engage with as many of the senses as you walk:** What can you hear, smell, see, and taste? Notice the air against your skin.
- **Beginner's eyes:** With each step, take each sensation with openness and curiosity, as though you were doing it for the first time.

Mindful Running

Release yourself from external distractions and daily pressures through the practice of mindful running.

- **Engage with as many of your five senses** as you can and leave the headphones at home.
- **Pay attention to the sensation of breathing:** Try focusing on breathing through your nose, as mouth breathing is related to the stress response.
- **Notice your thoughts and feelings with kindness and acceptance:** Try to reduce worrying about timings or tracking devices. If you find yourself ruminating or being critical, gently nudge your attention back to your breath instead of honing into the thoughts.
- **Hone into gratitude** of being able to physically run and making this time a priority.
- **Note how your body is reacting** as you get further into your run. Are you feeling any discomfort? Do you need to take a break or slow down, or do you want to challenge yourself a little more?
- **Reflect on how this running session made you feel:** Pay attention to how your heart rate slows, your breathing, and how your muscles feel as you stretch and cool down.
- **Celebrate this moment** and the work you have put into your physical health.

Yoga

Yoga combines physical poses, breathing practices, relaxation, and meditation. For many people, yoga is a self-discovery journey, bringing peace of mind and greater well-being. Consistent practice develops self-acceptance. Whatever your age or level of fitness, yoga is suitable for everyone. Through the practice of yoga, we can learn how to slow down and connect with our body and mind. Reset the body and mind with the *Mindful Movement Using Yoga* worksheet.

Chair Yoga

No matter how busy we are as dental professionals, we often have unexpected pockets of time, a few minutes here and there, where we can fit in physical movement. Chair yoga involves practising yoga sitting on a chair or standing, using a chair as support. This form of yoga was developed by Lakshmi Voelker-Binder in 1982. There are numerous benefits to chair yoga: improved muscle tone, better breathing habits, stress reduction, better sleep, and an improved sense of well-being. Try the *Yoga on the Dental Stool* worksheet when you are next working at your dental practice.

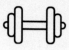

Mindful Movement Using Yoga

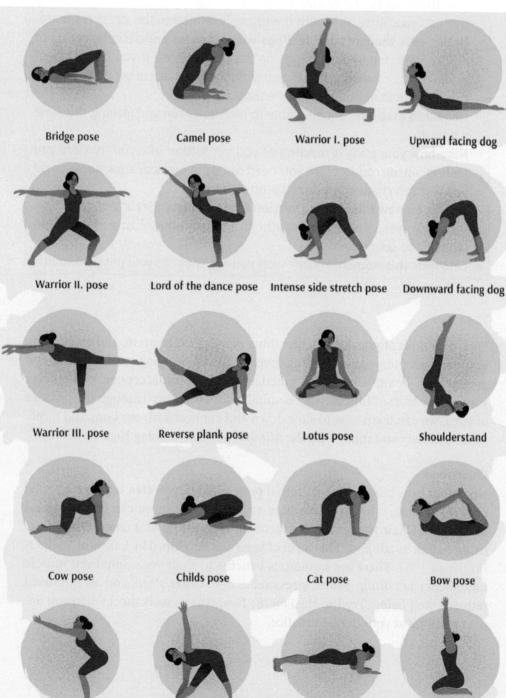

Bridge pose

Camel pose

Warrior I. pose

Upward facing dog

Warrior II. pose

Lord of the dance pose

Intense side stretch pose

Downward facing dog

Warrior III. pose

Reverse plank pose

Lotus pose

Shoulderstand

Cow pose

Childs pose

Cat pose

Bow pose

Chair

Extended triangle

Plank pose

Thunderbolt pose

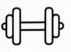

Mindful Movement Using Yoga

1. Choose a space that is free from clutter and distraction. If you like, light a candle or incense stick to help create a relaxing environment.

2. Select a yoga pose from the previous yoga illustration.

3. As you breathe in, go into your chosen yoga pose.

4. Connect with your breath and turn your attention inwards for several breaths.

5. Breathe deeply in this pose for several moments.

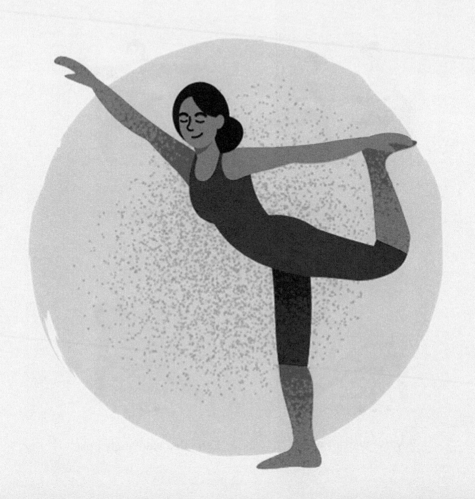

Yoga On The Dental Stool

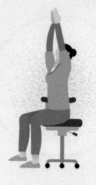

Sun salutations

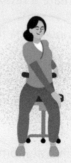

Seated spinal twist

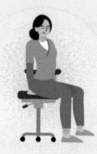

Chest opener

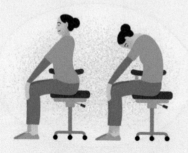

Cat- Cow pose

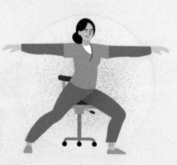

Warrior II. pose

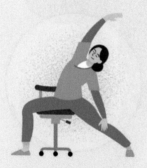

Reverse warrior pose

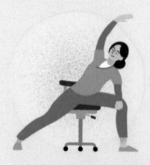

Extended side angle pose

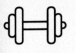

Yoga On The Dental Stool

Reset your body and mind with a simple breathing practice and these chair yoga poses that you can do in the clinic.

1. Start with sitting up straight. Lengthen your spine by imagining an invisible thread gently drawing you up through the crown of your head.

2. Become aware of your body. Note the points of contact, such as your bottom on the chair and your feet on the floor.

3. Tune into your breath. Become aware of the cool flow of air in your nostrils as you inhale and the warmed air as you exhale.

4. Take three deep, nourishing breaths. Feel the energising quality of every inhale and the complete release in every exhale.

5. Pick a pose and do this next. Poses can be done in a sequence, or you could concentrate on any pose you need right now.

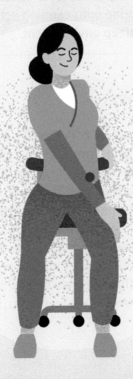

Restore with Sleep

Sleep and mood are closely connected. As dental professionals working so closely with patients, we can appreciate the impact of how reduced sleep hours may cause stress and irritability and often impact our following working day. This may spiral into a vicious cycle. Prioritising quality and consistent sleep is fundamental to building resilience – without this basic need, we struggle to optimally function. An adequate number of hours of sleep can enhance our psychological and physical well-being (Dinges et al. 1997). Furthermore, sleep problems, such as chronic insomnia, may increase our risk of developing mood disorders – for example, anxiety and depression (Breslau et al. 1996; Necklemann et al. 2007; Weissman et al. 1997). Following are sleep hygiene tips that can help us get better quality sleep.

Sleep Hygiene Practices

- **Sleep at the same time every night**, even on the weekends, as maintaining the timing of the body's internal clock can help you fall asleep and wake up more easily.
- **Expose yourself to light during the day** and limit light in the evening.
- **Avoid caffeine, alcohol, nicotine, and other chemicals** that interfere with sleep.
- **Avoid naps** close to your regular bedtime.
- **Avoid eating or exercising too soon** to bedtime.
- **Adopt a night time routine** with calming activities.
- **Create a comfortable sleep environment.**

Lessons from Blue Zones

Thinking about lifestyle factors collectively, across cultures, interesting research by Dan Buettner and Sam Skemp reports regions of the world where people statistically live longer and are healthier than the average, known as 'Blue Zones' (Buettner and Skemp 2016). Five 'Blue Zones' have been discussed: Okinawa (Japan), Sardinia (Italy), Nicoya (Costa Rica), Icaria (Greece), and Loma Linda (California, USA). Although their lifestyles differ slightly, below are seven lifestyle lessons from people living in Blue Zone regions. It is worth noting that much of what is spotlighted by these authors corroborates with the research in positive psychology on positive health protective factors: movement, sleep, nutrition, emotional regulation, meaning, and community.

1) **Incorporate natural movement:** Blue Zone inhabitants do this by living in environments that continuously nudge them into moving without thinking about it. We can incorporate this strategy through walking rather than driving wherever possible, using stairs, scheduling a hike with a friend to catch up rather than dinner, and playing outside with your pets and children.

2) **Have a sense of purpose.**

3) **Use strategies that help manage stress:** from mindfulness, colouring, and running to cooking a nutritious meal, find activities that help you downregulate and feel calmer.

4) **Eat until 80% full** rather than to excess each meal.

5) **Invite more vegetables and fruits into your diet:** people living in Blue Zones tend to enjoy mostly a plant-based diet and consume low amounts of meat.

6) **Priortise a good night's sleep.**

7) **Build a tribe that supports healthy behaviours:** Belonging to positive social and spiritual communities helps in feeling connected and supported in long-term healthy habits.

Summary

- A lifestyle change, with plenty of self-compassion, is required to create sustainable positive health.
- Nourish with eating a balanced diet and drinking plenty of water.
- Keeping the gut healthy with gut-friendly foods and drinks can help keep your brain healthy too.
- Replenish with increasing movement in your day, such as mindful walking at lunchtime, running, and practising chair yoga on the dental stool.
- Restore with good sleep hygiene practices.

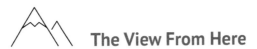 **The View From Here**

The 'L' of the PERLE Resilience Model acknowledges the importance of physical well-being in mental wellness. From nourishing our bodies with nutritious foods to replenishing with movement and restoring with sleep, if we want to have long, healthy dental careers, we need to make lifestyle shifts to support that longevity. Admittedly, this pillar is one that does not come so readily to me! I can quite easily get lost in writing and my tasks, completely forgoing scheduling in regular moments of physical care. However, making this pillar more prominent in my day to day adds so much to my sense of wellness. The hack I find helpful is to embed lifestyle in habits you already do – practise chair yoga in between patients, piggyback listening to your podcast with a walk, replace your sweet drawer with your favourite, nutritious snacks, or set an alarm for bedtime so you can schedule in 'me' time and your personalised wind down for a great night's rest.

References

Akkasheh, G., Kashani-Poor, Z., Tajabadi-Ebrahimi, M. et al. (2016). Clinical and metabolic response to probiotic administration in patients with major depressive disorder: a randomized, double-blind, placebo-controlled trial. *Nutrition* 32 (3): 315–320.

Breslau, N., Roth, T., Rosenthal, L., and Andreski, P. (1996). Sleep disturbance and psychiatric disorders: a longitudinal epidemiological study of young adults. *Biological Psychiatry* 39: 411–418.

Buettner, D. and Skemp, S. (2016). Blue Zones: lessons from the world's longest lived. *American Journal of Lifestyle Medicine* 10 (5): 318–321.

Dinges, D.F., Pack, F., Williams, K. et al. (1997). Cumulative sleepiness, mood disturbance, and psychomotor vigilance performance decrements during a week of sleep restricted to 4–5 hours per night. *Sleep* 20: 267–277.

Hilimire, M.R., DeVylder, J.E., and Forestell, C.A. (2015). Fermented foods, neuroticism, and social anxiety: an interaction model. *Psychiatry Research* 228 (2): 203–208.

Hyde, A.L., Maher, J.P., and Elavsky, S. (2013). Enhancing our understanding of physical activity and wellbeing with a lifespan perspective. *International Journal of Wellbeing* 3.

Jorde, R., Sneve, M., Figenschau, Y. et al. (2008). Effects of vitamin D supplementation on symptoms of depression in overweight and obeese subjects: randomized double blind trial. *Journal of Internal Medicine* 264: 599–609.

Messaoudi, M., Lalonde, R., Violle, N. et al. (2011a). Assessment of psychotropic-like properties of a probiotic formulation (Lactobacillus helveticus R0052 and Bifidobacterium longum R0175) in rats and human subjects. *British Journal of Nutrition* 105 (5): 755–764.

Messaoudi, M., Violle, N., Bisson, J.F. et al. (2011b). Beneficial psychological effects of a probiotic formulation (Lactobacillus helveticus R0052 and Bifidobacterium longum R0175) in healthy human volunteers. *Gut Microbes* 2 (4): 256–261.

Neckelmann, D., Mykletun, A., and Dahl, A.A. (2007). Chronic insomnia as a risk factor for developing anxiety and depression. *Sleep* 30: 873–880.

Rees, K., Takeda, A., Martin, N. et al. (2019). Mediterranean-style diet for the primary and secondary prevention of cardiovascular disease. *Cochrane Database of Systematic Reviews* 3.

Ulmer, C.S., Stetson, B.A., and Salmon, P.G. (2010). Mindfulness and acceptance are associated with exercise maintenance in YMCA exercisers. *Research Behavior and Therapy* 48 (8): 805–809.

Weissman, M.M., Greenwald, S., Niño-Murcia, G., and Dement, W.C. (1997). The morbidity of insomnia uncomplicated by psychiatric disorders. *General Hospital Psychiatry* 19: 245–250.

10

Positive Work Environments

CHAPTER OVERVIEW

- Understanding the role of environment at work in building greater resilience and well-being
- Well-being ideas for dental teams
- Benefits of High-Quality Connections
- Neuroscience of High-Quality Connections
- Pathways to building High-Quality Connections in dentistry
- Understanding character strengths
- Benefits of strengths approach in dentistry
- Applying strengths with patients and at home.

People do not leave jobs, they leave toxic work environments.

—Anonymous

The environment in which we work as dental professionals matters enormously to our mental well-being. Negative work environments in dentistry, with behaviours such as bullying and rudeness, have wide-spanning downstream impacts on the dental professional, the team, patients, and also our personal relationships at home. When we experience rudeness and incivility from a work colleague, it triggers a stress response and the amygdala hijack we discussed in Chapter 1. The consequences of this stress response include reduced thinking abilities and the inability to problem solve because we are lost mulling over the rude comments. We are less likely to seek help or share learnings from failures with our team, as we are operating from a space of fear. We spend so much time at work, and so if we are surrounded by toxic work cultures, no matter how much we focus on the other pillars of resilience, thriving at work becomes that much harder.

Conversely, a positive working environment encourages us to feel happier at work and connected to our team, to be more productive, and to be much more equipped to perform as a dental professional efficiently. We feel

Resilience and Well-being for Dental Professionals, First Edition. Mahrukh Khwaja.
© 2023 John Wiley & Sons Ltd. Published 2023 by John Wiley & Sons Ltd.
Companion website: www.wiley.com/go/khwaja-resilience-dentistry

psychologically safe – that is, comfortable to bring our authentic selves to work without fear of reprimand, punishment, or discrimination. We feel safe to share concerns and have positive discussions.

The 'E' of the PERLE Resilience Model centres on exactly these components. This chapter hones in on an environment at work that is compassionate, positive, and centred on well-being and allows us to perform in optimal states.

Positive Practices for Teams: Nurturing Positive Work Environments

Positive teams grow positive work cultures. Here are suggestions on how dental principals and practice managers can nurture positive work cultures, underpinned by well-being principles.

- **Morning and afternoon check in huddles:** Questions include enquiring how each team member is feeling, their energy levels, if they need any support for their tasks, and what's going well
- **Zero tolerance for disruptive behaviour**, such as rudeness, bullying, and discrimination.
- **Mini breaks** during the work day for High-Quality Connections, taking mindful deep breaths, and rest. Encouraging break during lunchtime, rather than working throughout, for example, going for a walk instead of having lunch whilst writing notes/referrals.
- **Designated mental well-being champion** for the team, trained in mental health first aid – to spot early signs of poor mental health and provide guidance on support. The mental well-being champion may also organise team-bonding days/events to encourage healthy living and gather feedback to inform future initiatives for the team.
- **Protected time to complete well-being and resilience training annually**.
- **Ability for staff to take holidays** for recovery, rest, and restoration.
- **Regular acts of kindness at** work.
- **Celebrating team wins,** as well as staff recognition for small and big.
- **Staff lunch dates** where the team gets together for catching up and connecting.
- **Regular and optional socials** outside work.
- **Organising a team fundraising activity,** such as a charity run.
- **Spotlighting a well-being idea** for every team meeting agenda.
- **Control over workload** and clinical diary: Dental professionals having the autonomy to book patient treatments, review targets regularly, and minimise a culture of double-booking appointment slots for dental emergencies or extending the work day. Consider zoning appointments for emergencies.
- **Protected time for referrals/admin** in the patient diary.
- **Mentorship and coaching.**
- **Debriefing** after incidents.

The physical environment within the dental practice also impacts our well-being and productivity. Dental principals can bake well-being principles into the design of their practice. This could be through:

- **Well-being notice board** with well-being tips, the *Mental Wellness Check-in* (see Chapter 3), and staff recognition through posting gratitude and compliments
- **Thoughts box** for staff to anonymously document feelings
- **Boosting natural light** as much as possible, through use of windows
- **Avoiding harsh fluorescent lighting:** when the lighting is too harsh it can cause eye strain or headaches
- **Ergonomic chairs**
- **Encouraging use of loupes** for clinical procedures
- **Dedicated staff room**
- **Air con**.

In the next sections, we explore in depth two key ways dental professionals can be active in creating positive work environments: through improving relationships at work by boosting High-Quality Connections, and increasing engagement by activating our top strengths with patients and the team.

High-Quality Connections

The practice of dentistry can be a lonely endeavour. We may face a busy patient diary, with emergency appointments, referrals, and juggling record keeping in between difficult treatments, with little respite. It can be very easy to not prioritise our relationships at work and suffer from isolation in the process. However, examining our physiology when we experience loneliness shines new light on this topic: loneliness puts us in a 'stressed' state, with the body releasing stress hormones, such as cortisol. And as we established in Chapter 1, chronic stress states impact both our mental and physical well-being. One large meta-analysis of 70 studies with more than three million participants showed loneliness had a significant effect on mortality, which has been shown to be similar to effects to smoking 15 cigarettes day (Holt-Lunstad et al. 2015).

The key to transforming the dental environment, and an effective antidote to loneliness in dentistry, is to build and nurture positive relationships. We can do this through increasing our High-Quality Connections (HQCs) at work. HQCs can be defined as very short interactions, *even seconds*, that are positive, characterised by positive regard (warmth towards the other person), vitality (feeling energised and connected), and mutuality (finding common ground) (Dutton and Heaphy 2003). These micro-moments of connection should be considered the same as any health behaviour: crucial in survival but also for us to thrive. HQCs make us feel more open and alive. They boost our levels of positive emotions, and as Fredrickson's Broaden-and-Build Theory describes (see Chapter 3), our thinking is broadened as a result, and we build important psychological and psychical resources that can support us.

It has long been established that as dental professionals we benefit from prioritising connection with our patients before starting treatment, in order to build trusting relationships and avoid litigation. What is not featured, however, is the sheer possibilities of these HQCs to boost our psychological well-being. We have moments upon moments, meeting numerous patients, to top up our levels of HQCs.

Benefits of HQC for Dental Professionals and Teams

- Improve the health of dental professionals, such as their thinking (Carmelli et al. 2015), reduced negative arousal, memory, improved job satisfaction, and immune system (Heaphy and Dutton 2008).
- May facilitate dental professionals' ability to be resilient, through managing stressors effectively at work and adapting to change (Stephens et al. 2013).
- Nurture psychological safety and trust (Carmeli and Gittell 2009; Carmeli et al. 2009).
- Improve team processes, including team learning from failures.

Neuroscience of Connection

Micro-moments of connection with our patients, work colleagues, and loved ones are no ordinary moments. Barbara Fredrickson describes that 'a powerful back-and-forth union of energy springs up between the two of you, like an electric charge' (Fredrickson 2014). Brain imaging studies show that we oscillate and resonate chemicals, such as oxytocin, dopamine, and serotonin, when we share HQCs with others. When speaking with work colleagues and patients you know well, it sets up pleasure centres and reward centres, firing motor neurons in your social–emotional centre, making you feel more connected to the other person and safer. These brain regions light up because you are excited talking to the other person, and you also have a the same effect on the other person's brain.

Pathways for Building HQCs in Dentistry

There are several pathways to building HQCs in dentistry, interacting both with our patients and team. We focus on four pathways: mindful listening, team gratitude, positive communication, and mentoring. Drawing from the research from Dutton and others, these pathways create an environment at work that honours respect and kindness and increases our capacity to be more helpful to our team and patients.

Mindful Listening

An important part of teamwork, as well as positive relationships with our patients, is effective communication. Mindful listening can play a significant role in this. This is a way of listening with our full attention, without judgement, criticism, or interruption. Mindful listening techniques can help us truly understand what our patients, colleagues, and loved ones are saying. It can also help us build trust.

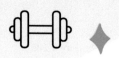

Mindful Listening

With this mindful practice, we listen with intention and focus on the other person. Giving someone your full attention in conversation is not easy, but it is a skill we can practice and hone. Try this mindful listening exercise with a dental colleague.

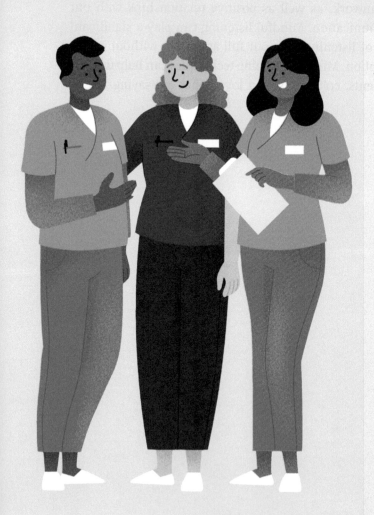

- For the next 10 minutes, when you are in conversation with your colleague, place your entire focus on that person.

- Instead of thinking what to say next, use non-verbal gestures such as nodding, maintaining eye contact, and smiling. This will to encourage other people to express their thoughts.

- Reflect back words and emotions expressed.

- Practise compassion when listening.

- When you notice your mind wander, gently nudge your attention back to what is being said.

Team Gratitude

Think About It

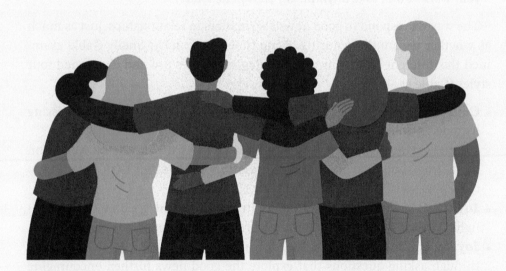

Building a culture of gratitude at work is a great way of nurturing stronger, more resilient teams, and positive relationships with our colleagues. Here are some suggestions on how you can foster a gratitude culture:

- In your team meeting, go around each team member sharing a gratitude point from your day. This could be something that went well during your clinic or a compliment a patient made. Big or small.
- Create a gratitude board – with a space to share positive gratitude points about other work colleagues.
- Have regular gratitude conversations.
- Celebrate each other's successes.
- Practise acts of kindness with your team.
- Praise each other for positive progress.
- Write thank you notes.

Positive Communication

HQCs often begin with asking the right questions. With our patients and work colleagues we can ask:

- **Questions that unearth common ground:** *What is your favourite hobby outside of work? What has been your most enjoyable holiday? What are you most looking forward to in the next three months?*
- **Questions that portray genuine interest in the other person:** *What gives you joy at work? What are you most grateful for this week? What went well for you this week? What has been the most meaningful part of your work week?*
- **Questions that offer help to colleagues:** *In what ways can I help you with your work? Can I take anything off your plate today?*

The way we respond to good news also matters in relationships, just as much as whether we are there during trying times. Researcher Shelly Gable examined the different communication strategies couples use and discovered four styles (Gable et al. 2006):

- **Conversation killer:** This refers to stopping the conversation progressing by moving onto another topic altogether.
- **Conversation hijacker:** This style refers to hijacking the conversation by talking about the good news in relation to us rather than listening to our colleagues' good news.
- **Joy thief:** In this style, all of the negatives around the good news are highlighted instead of revelling in the joy of the good news.
- **Joy multiplier:** This style focuses on delving into the good news fully through asking questions that explore the good news further, encouraging an upwards spiral of positive emotions between your colleague and yourself.

As you may have guessed, the joy multiplier is the most effective way of communicating positively with our work colleagues! We can develop this skill by showing our curiosity and engagement by asking questions; using supportive language, positive non-verbal cues, and energy; and expressing positive emotion.

Mentoring and Coaching

Having a mentor or coach in dentistry has the powerful potential of reducing isolation through providing support in a safe environment as well as increasing the important HQCs. All the features of HQCs are generated through interactions with a coach: an upwards spiral of positive emotions, feeling energised, and a sense of common ground. It gives dental professionals the opportunities to delve into concerns, challenges, solutions, goals, and purpose. All dental professionals are growing and developing and hence could benefit from mentoring. Teams could create a mentoring culture, where senior staff could help mentees by talking through cases, sharing their own challenges and how they overcame them, and aiding in increasing autonomy for the mentee in learning for themselves and discovering their own direction in dentistry. And if mentoring is not readily available at work, we can look to coaches within the industry.

Engagement at Work

> *A meaningful life is using your signature strengths and virtues in the service of something much larger than you are.*
>> —Martin Seligman, psychologist, professor, founder of the positive psychology movement and the PERMA theory, researcher on well-being

When we are burnt out as dental professionals, we experience deep emotional exhaustion, cynicism towards work, and inefficiency. Work engagement is the converse of this: we feel **energised, absorbed at work, and dedicated to mastery of skills**. Indeed, research shows engaged employees are less likely to experience burnout and more likely to be attached to and satisfied with their organisations. One route to increasing our sense of engagement at work is to double down on our strengths, both with patients and outside the clinic.

Studies show that adopting a strengths-based approach is a more effective generator for change; helps us enhance our social relationships, build better coping strategies during challenges, and reduce depressive symptoms; and is good for the bottom line (Sin and Lyubomirsky 2009; Linley 2008). The way this works is through raising our levels of positive emotions through getting us into a psychological state of 'flow', boosting our engagement, and inviting more meaning and resilience. Doubling down on strengths makes a lot of sense: it is good for us, our patients, our relationships, and organisations we work for.

What are Character Strengths?

Character strengths refer to the authentic, positive aspects of our personality that help us shine in life. Understanding what we are good at can help us answer what we stand for and how we can contribute for the greater good. Using our strengths every day can help us feel more engaged with life and

WISDOM	**Creativity** Showing originality, adaptability and ingenuity	**Curiosity** Openness to new ideas and keenness to explore	**Judgment** Open-mindedness and the ability to think critically	**Love of Learning** Mastering new skills and gathering knowledge	**Perspective** Providing wise counsel and taking a big-picture view
COURAGE	**Bravery** Acting with conviction in the face of challenges and despite doubts or fears	**Amend to Perseverance** Showing tenacity in achieving goals despite obstacles, discouragements, or disappointments	**Honesty** Acting with authenticity and integrity	**Zest** Approaching life with vitality, enthusiasm and energy	
HUMANITY	**Love** Experiencing and valuing close, loving relationships with others	**Kindness** Showing generosity, compassion and altruism			**Social Intelligence** Understanding the motives and feelings of self and others
JUSTICE	**Teamwork** Demonstrating loyalty and social responsibility; collaborating with others to achieve a goal			**Fairness** Treating everyone equally and fairly, without bias	**Leadership** Organising and encouraging others to get things done and achieve a shared vision.
TEMPERANCE		**Forgiveness** Acceptance of others' shortcomings and being willing to give people a second chance	**Humility** Letting one's accomplishments speak for themselves, without seeking attention or recognition	**Prudence** Being careful and cautious; not taking unnecessary risks	**Self-Regulation** Showing discipline and self-control
TRANSCENDENCE	**Appreciation of Beauty & Excellence** Feeling awe and wonder about the world and the skill of others	**Gratitude** Feeling blessed and expressing thanks	**Hope** Optimism for the future	**Humour** Showing playfulness and lightheartedness	**Spirituality** Feeling a sense of purpose and meaning in life and acknowledging your place in the universe

Figure 10.1 VIA classification of character strengths (Seligman et al. 2004).

bring the best of who we are to our everyday. Even when managing depression, positive psychotherapy interventions that include strengths report excellent clinical findings (Seligman et al. 2006).

The VIA (Values in Action) Institute of Character is a not-for-profit organisation that was founded in response to the research by Seligman and colleagues into strengths. The researchers examined strengths across different cultures and countries, collating 24 character strengths with six overall virtues: wisdom, courage, humanity, justice, temperance, and transcendence (see Figure 10.1).

Strengths amongst Medical Professionals

A strengths-based approach in dentistry (or even more broadly within health-care) is currently uncharted territory. However, there is growing interest in this area. One recent literature review examined character strengths profiles of medical students and doctors, specifically their impact on well-being and work engagement (Huber et al. 2020). The authors reported that strengths of com-passion, courage, altruism, and benevolence were conveyed most often. From the VIA character strengths profile, the strengths of fairne, honesty, kindness, and teamwork were reported to be especially key for medical professionals. Students interested in paediatrics reported higher levels of kindness, whereas students interested in surgery reported more bravery. The positive impact of applying character strengths to work and increasing well-being is in line with numerous studies on strengths and well-being (Govindji and Linley 2007; Littman-Ovadia and Steger 2010; Seligman 2011; Harzer and Ruch 2012, 2013). The authors advised promoting self-awareness and character building among medical professionals as a beneficial strategy in boosting clinician well-being, work engagement, and improved patient-centred care.

Using Strengths in Dentistry

Drawing on the science of strengths, utilising our key strengths in our every-day in new and engaging ways can boost our well-being and build resilience. We can even use strengths to help us overcome challenges. In Table 10.1 are some examples of how we can activate our strengths at work and outside.

Table 10.1 Activating strengths.

Character strength	How to activate this strength
Teamwork	• Find new ways to contribute to the team: this may be asking your work colleagues if they need assistance or mentoring. • Organise team bonding days. • Mediate a team discussion and attempt to achieve consensus on a conflicting issue. Whatever the result, aim to understand more about the different views of each team member.
Leadership	• Lead an activity at work, encouraging members who rarely speak to share their opinions. • Mediate conflict at work by encouraging others to share their thoughts and spotlight problem solving. Set an emphatic, respectful, and open-minded tone for the discussion. • Reflect on different ways you can improve your leadership style. Ask your team members for their input.
Gratitude	• Reflect on three past challenges in dentistry and three good things they led to. • Reminisce your best moments of recognition, achievement, praise, and connection. • Show gratitude to a colleague who makes your day better. • Share gratitude during a team meeting.
Kindness	• Do three random acts of kindness per week at work. • Do a random act of kindness for someone you do not know.
Love of learning	• Identify topics on which you can share knowledge with dental peers. • Start a new course. • Arrange a teach-learn date with a friend. • Take learning breaks during the day.
Appreciation of beauty	• Notice natural beauty everyday by going on a nature walk. • Listen to moving piece of music. • Appreciate a beautiful piece of art or poetry.
Love	• Arrange a date with your partner that celebrates both of your signature strengths. • Focus on implicit motives of loved ones rather than behaviours. • Explore and appreciate strengths of loved ones.
Spirituality	• Schedule time to meditate. • Sit down, light a candle, and journal. • Read your favourite spiritual text. • Volunteer at a charity that is meaningful. • Connect with nature.

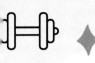

Discover Your Strengths

1. Fill out the free, scientific strengths assessment online at www.viacharacter.org. This will highlight your top five strengths. Write these down.

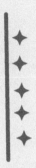

2. How are you currently using these strengths with patients and outside the clinic? Which of your strengths support you the most in doing what you love?

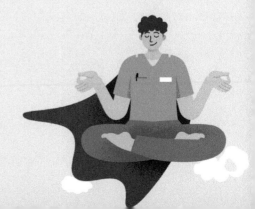

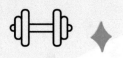

Discover Your Strengths

3. Strengths can be used to overcome difficulties and take positive action to move forward. Which of these strengths have you used to overcome a challenge?

4. Think of ways you can activate your strengths and use them in new and engaging ways during your week. What might you need to change to make it happen?

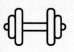

Discover Your Strengths

5. What unexplored strengths would you like to develop?

6. What goal could you set that would encourage you to use your strengths more with patients and in your personal life? What small steps can you take to move forward?

Discovering Optimal Use of Strengths

In the same way strengths can be underused, they may also be overused, causing a myriad of negative impacts on oneself, such as overworking, or on others. Dental professionals high in appreciation of beauty and excellence, for example, may find themselves constantly upholding unrealistic standards in dentistry or in their relationships. Often when we are overusing our character strengths, we have brought the strength to the wrong situation or have misinterpreted the surrounding context. They key is finding your optimal use: **the right combination of strengths, to the right degree, and in the right situation**. The following self-reflection questions will help you work out your strengths sweet spot.

> - Reflect on what it feels like when you overuse your top strengths. How does it impact yourself and others?
> - What does it feel like when you underuse your strengths? How does it impact yourself and others?
> - Consider a recent challenge at work or a stressor. Which character strengths were you underusing and which were you overusing?
> - In situations in which you find yourself upset or irritated by others, are you overplaying or underplaying any of your character strengths?

Achieving Flow

Achieving more moments of psychological flow not only feels exhilarating but also helps build greater well-being and resilience. Athletes regularly use flow to their advantage to help them win games, stay focused, and compete at the highest levels. But flow is for everyone. Our flow activities could be playing a sport, writing, poetry, teaching, mountain climbing, hiking, photography, playing an instrument, painting, or upcycling furniture. We could also experience flow at work; for example, whilst composite bonding, facial aesthetics, or orthodontic treatment. Making time for more moments of flow are the moments in life that will bolster us against stressors and create a life that is rich and meaningful.

It is very easy not to give our hobbies much importance. However, we all know that time is a precious commodity, and how we spend it is important. Instead of wearing overworking as a badge of honour, championing our leisure time as much as our work time will benefit our lives.

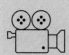

Learning From Movies

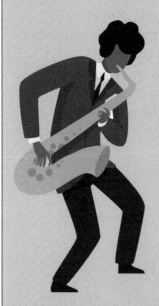

A Case Study: **Soul** *by Disney Pixar*

Disney Pixar's movie *Soul* beautifully brings to life what flow looks and feels like. It tells the story of Joe, a band teacher, whose life has not quite panned out the way he expected. His true love is playing jazz music. But it is not until he travels to another realm to help someone else work out their true purpose that he discovers what it means it have soul. When Joe talks about his passion for jazz and starts playing, he has an out-of-body experience. He is transformed to another dimension, where it is just him and his music. The feeling of time changes. This film expertly illustrates the experiential quality of flow experiences, the altered perception of time, the effortlessness, the high concentration and melting together of action and consciousness. These conditions are drawn from the research by Mihaly Csikszentmihalyi and his work on Flow Theory (Csikszentmihalyi 1990). Csikszentmihalyi describes flow as 'a state in which people are so involved in an activity that nothing else seems to matter; the experience is so enjoyable that people will continue to do it even at great cost, for the sheer sake of doing it'. This movie also poignantly captures the connection between flow and well-being: the experience of jazz brings Joe tremendous happiness, meaning, and purpose in life. What activities bring about flow in you?

Key Takeaways from Flow Research

- Everyone can achieve flow, young and old.
- We need uninterrupted time to concentrate on a task to experience flow.
- Flow experiences can be increased by intentionally engaging with them everyday.
- Flow contributes to our happiness

Summary

- Positive work environments support our psychological well-being and resilience.
- Two pathways include HQCs and using our strengths at work.
- HQCs can be strengthened within dental teams through mindful listening, team gratitude, positive communication, and mentoring.
- Character strengths are positive parts of our personality that impact how we think, feel, and act.
- Use strengths profilers to work out your top five strengths; for example, VIA profiler (www.viacharacter.org).
- Flow increases well-being and happiness.
- For flow to be achieved, we need uninterrupted time.

 The View From Here

Positive work environments allow us to live optimally rather than just at baseline. Having worked in both NHS and private settings as a UK dentist for 12 years and coached many dental professionals, the impact of toxic work environments (bullying, incivility, critical management styles) on our wellness is not lost on me. Furthermore, there are the downstream impacts of negative work environment on our personal relationships. The antidote is creating dental environments that allow for us to thrive – ones that champion our well-being.

Thinking about our environment at work, and how we can be active change makers in creating positive work cultures, prioritising our relationships and using our strengths, has enormous 360-degree benefits on our quality of life in dentistry. The 'E' of PERLE celebrates this important aspect and reminds us to take action in building a positive climate in the dental practice. Dental principals and practice managers have a multitude of options in really doubling down on well-being through adopting simple well-being strategies, from adopting a well-being champion to regular check-ins using the *Mental Wellness Check-in* and promoting rest breaks and an open-door policy to foster safe spaces to share concerns. At the individual level, dental professionals can boost relationships at work through seeking HQCs with patients and the team. Furthermore, dental professionals can reflect upon and identify core strengths and apply these strengths when working with patients as well as in their interpersonal relationships.

The foundation of every dental team is great relationships at work. And through building upon a solid foundation of well-being that supports every team member, principals and practice managers are much more likely to retain staff long term, prevent absenteeism and presenteeism, and boost team morale. A positive environment within the dental clinic goes even further than that: it nurtures a thriving team. Now that's something to really celebrate and work towards. A simple yet effective way we can lean into this every day is to ask ourselves: How can I contribute to creating a kinder climate at work today? It is through these small actions, day by day, that we make a big difference to our collective happiness. And where work cultures are sadly embedded with toxicity, to leave and seek opportunities where our resilience levels can be replenished.

References

Carmeli, A. and Gittell, J.R. (2009). High quality relationships, psychological safety and learning from failures in work organizations. *Journal of Organizational Behavior* 30: 709–729.

Carmeli, A., Brueller, D., and Dutton, J.E. (2009). Learning behaviors in the workplace: the role of high-quality interpersonal relationships and psychological safety. *Systems Research and Behavioral Science* 26 (1): 81–98.

Carmeli, A., Dutton, J.E., and Hardin, A.E. (2015). Respect as an engine for new ideas: linking respectful engagement, relational information processing and creativity among employees and teams. *Human Relations Journal* 68 (6): 1021–1047.

Csikszentmihalyi, M. (1990). *Flow: The Psychology of Optimal Experience*, 1e. New York: Harper & Row.

Dutton, J.E. and Heaphy, E. (2003). The power of high-quality connections. In: *Positive Organizational Scholarship: Foundations of a New Discipline* (ed. K.S. Cameron, J.E. Dutton and R.E. Quinn). San Francisco: Berrett-Koehler.

Fredrickson, B. (2014). *Love 2.0: Creating Happiness and Health in Moments of Connection*. New York: Plume.

Gable, S.L., Gonzaga, G.C., and Strachman, A. (2006). Will you be there for me when things go right? Supportive responses to positive event disclosures. *Journal of Personality and Social Psychology* 91 (5): 904.

Govindji, R. and Linley, P.A. (2007). Strengths use, self-concordance and well-being: implications for strengths coaching and coaching psychologists. *International Coaching Psychology Review* 2: 143–153.

Harzer, C. and Ruch, W. (2012). When the job is a calling: the role of applying one's signature strengths at work. *Journal of Positive Psychology* 7: 362–371.

Harzer, C. and Ruch, W. (2013). The application of signature character strengths and positive experiences at work. *Journal of Happiness Studies* 14: 965–983.

Heaphy, E.D. and Dutton, J.E. (2008). Positive social interactions and the human body at work: linking organizations and physiology. *Academy of Management Review* 33 (1): 137–162.

Holt-Lunstad, J., Smith, T.B., Baker, M. et al. (2015). Loneliness and social isolation as risk factors for mortality: a meta-analytic review. *Perspectives on Psychological Science* 10 (2): 227–237. https://doi.org/10.1177/1745691614568352.

Huber, A., Strecker, C., Kachel, T. et al. (2020). Character strengths profiles in medical professionals and their impact on well-being. *Frontiers in Psychology* 11: 566728.

Linley, P.A. (2008). *Average to A+: Realising Strengths in Yourself and Others*. Coventry, UK: CAPP Press.

Littman-Ovadia, H. and Steger, M.F. (2010). Character strengths and well-being among volunteers and employees: toward an integrative model. *Journal of Positive Psychology* 5: 419–430.

Seligman, M.E.P. (2011). *Flourish: A Visionary New Understanding of Happiness and Wellbeing*. New York: Free Press.

Seligman, M.E., Park, N., and Peterson, C. (2004). The Values in Action (VIA) classification of character strengths. *Ricerche di Psicologia* 27: 63–78.

Seligman, M.E., Rashid, T., and Parks, A.C. (2006). Positive psychotherapy. *American Psychologist* 61 (8): 774.

Sin, N.L. and Lyubomirsky, S. (2009). Enhancing well-being and alleviating depressive symptoms with positive psychology interventions: a practice-friendly meta-analysis. *Journal of Clinical Psychology* 65 (5): 467–487.

Stephens, J.P., Heaphy, E.D., Carmeli, A. et al. (2013). Relationship quality and virtuousness: emotional carrying capacity as a source of individual and team resilience. *Journal of Applied Behavioral Science* 49: 13–41.

11

Work–Life Harmony

CHAPTER OVERVIEW

- Psychology of time
- Measure how you spend your time
- Nurturing work–life harmony
- Well-being, play, and dentistry
- Social media and digital well-being.

> *The key is not to prioritise what's on your schedule, but to schedule your priorities.*
>
> —Stephen Covey, author on habits of successful people

Are you constantly short of time? Do you find that you run out of time to study, socialise, go to the gym, or to do the things that matter to you the most? Our lives are busy, often packed to the brim with a never-ending list of to-do items. Capitalist culture puts inordinate value on productivity. Throw in more time spent on our phones since the rise of social media and apps, and this has resulted in the general trend of many of us feeling even busier than before. We are in a time crunch.

Exactly *how* we spend our time matters for both our professional and personal lives. Time is so significant that psychologists have coined special terms to describe this time crunch, *time famine*, starving for more time to do everything. The opposite interestingly is coined as *time affluence*, a metaphorical type of wealth where we have the time to do the things we long to do.

In this chapter, we examine the science of time, research insights on creating a better work–life balance for us, the importance of play over productivity alone, and digital well-being. The latter has massive drains to our time but, as with any tool, boundaries can benefit us.

Resilience and Well-being for Dental Professionals, First Edition. Mahrukh Khwaja.
© 2023 John Wiley & Sons Ltd. Published 2023 by John Wiley & Sons Ltd.
Companion website: www.wiley.com/go/khwaja-resilience-dentistry

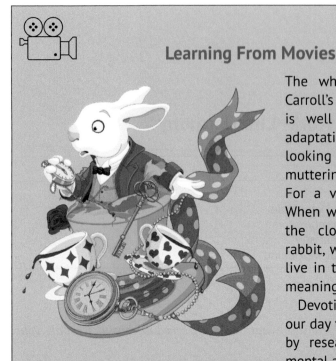

Learning From Movies

The white rabbit in Lewis Carroll's Alice in Wonderland is well known in Disney's adaptation for constantly looking at his watch and muttering, 'I'm late! I'm late! For a very important date!' When we become a slave to the clock, like the white rabbit, we lose our ability to live in the moment. We lose meaning and richness in life.

Devoting a good portion of our day to idling is backed up by research to benefit our mental and physical health as well as improve our creativity, relationships, and happiness levels. Author of How to Be Idle Tom Hodgkinson despises clocks. And his act of rebellion is idling – the act of taking the scenic route, long and happy conversations well into the wee hours, hanging out with friends doing nothing in particular, taking long naps, and daydreaming. He argues that if we neglect that part of life, we run the risk of overworking (Hodgkinson 2005).

Psychology of Time

Have you ever asked yourself, what is time? And how does culture impact our time use? Our culture does indeed impact how we use time. We have 'clock time' and within that a monochronic or polychronic time system. Monochronic time is where one activity or task is carried out at a time. Countries that utilise monochronic time include much of the Western world. Interestingly, monochronic time gets its roots from the Industrial Revolution, where the labour force had somewhere specific to be at each hour and minute of the day to meet large-scale factory production. Polychronic time is the opposite to monochronic; cultures where people on the whole view time as a more fluid concept, going with the flow of time rather than strictly following a time schedule.

Our Time Perspective

We are born time travellers. We relive our past memories, ground ourselves in the present, and anticipate future rewards. And how naturally we can travel back and forth makes a significant difference in how we succeed in life and how happy we are whilst we are living it. Out attitude towards time, whether we have a bias towards getting stuck in the past, live in the moment, or are constantly future-orientated, can predict numerous constructs, from our dental career to our well-being and happiness. In fact, psychologist Philip Zimbardo's pivotal research in the field of time goes one step further: our attitude towards time is just as defining as key personality traits, for example, optimism or sociability. It influences many of our emotions, motives, decisions, and actions (Zimbardo and Boyd 2008).

The way we use our time can give us meaningful direction, greater health, a more successful dental career, and more enjoyment in our relationships. Research on time explores how we each have an individual perspective on time, known as *time perspective*, thinking about the past, present, and future. Understanding our current time perspective and that of others is really crucial to our well-being – the idea is simple but has consequences on our relationships and on the world that are fundamental.

All individuals have a bias towards a particular time perspective. This bias is often learned in childhood. The factors that influence our time perspective include our family, friends, and role models, culture, geography, climate, religion, social class, educational level, and political and economic stability. Individualistic societies ('me focused'), such as common Western societies, tend to be future focused, whilst collectivistic societies ('we focused') invest more in the past. Our income also has an effect, with poorer communities tending to live more in the present. The crucial point to note, however, is that we can all change our time perspective.

Zimbardo describes five key types of time perspective. These are summarised in Table 11.1, along with the research findings according to each time perspective.

Table 11.1 Types of time perspective.

Time perspective	Research findings	Overusing this time perspective…
Past-positive; focus on positives thinking about the past, for example, reliving fond childhood memories.	• High levels correlate with greater happiness, high self-esteem, friendliness. • Past-positive, present-pleasure, and future-orientated related to positive social relationships. This may be due to reminiscing on positive times, living in the moment, and including people in a future you are creating.	• No negatives in the research for this perspective.
Past-negative; focus on negatives when thinking about the past, for example, regrets, missed opportunities.	• High levels linked to trait anxiety, depression, and aggression. • Holman and Zimbardo (2009) found that a past negative bias was correlated with low support and high conflict with family and friends. The authors suggested this may be due to individuals feeling trapped with resentful thoughts and unable to forgive others.	• Risk of depression. • Tips to moderate: reconstruct past negative experiences by discovering hidden positive elements; insert new slides in memory tray rather than reliving negative; recollect recent positive emotions. • Research shows memory of past is fragile and distorted and unreliable.
Present-pleasure; focus on grounding ourselves in the present moment. We prioritise seeking pleasure. Known in psychology as present-hedonism.	• Moderately high levels result in greater well-being and resilience. • At the extreme end; novelty seeking, aggression, alcohol and drug use.	• When overused, may find it difficult to delay gratification and get tasks done. • Tip to moderate: set 20-minute chunks of time to work followed by a pleasurable activity.

Table 11.1 (Continued)

Time perspective	Research findings	Overusing this time perspective...
Present-fatalistic; a belief that our life is already mapped out for us and we do not have any control over its course. Known in psychology as present-fatalism.	• High levels linked to high aggression, trait anxiety, depression. • Mello and Worrell (2006) found that people with this time perspective had much lower academic success than people with a future-orientated perspective, perhaps due to procrastination.	• Avoid putting yourself outside your comfort zone and learn new things due to a belief everything is predetermined; 'fixed mindset'. • Tip to moderate: adopt a 'growth mindset' approach.
Future; focus on the future, for example, engaging with health-related behaviours that have no immediate impact but offer a future benefit. Work towards long-term bigger rewards instead settling for short-term quick ones.	• Moderately high levels correlate with greater success due to the ability to delay gratification. • High levels correlated with sacrificing family time, friend time, fun time, personal indulgences, hobbies, and sleep for success, living for work, achievement, and control.	• Anxiety about future, lack of enjoyment in present. • Sacrifice friends, family. • Locked into a time crunch. • Overinvested in the future. • Tips to moderate: do less, not more; make conscious choices about what matters most; reserve at least one weekend day as a workless day; disconnect; try to minimise intrusion of work into your home life.

Think About It

Time Perspective on Our Decision-Making

How does time perspective influence our decision-making and actions? Use this flow diagram to think about your decision-making. Which time orientation do you tend to use the most?

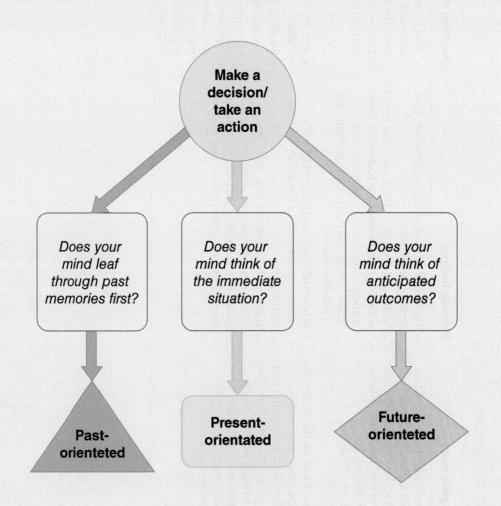

Measure Your Well-being

Measure your time perspective using the Zimbardo Time Perspective Inventory:

www.thetimeparadox.com/zimbardo-time-perspective-inventory/.

Is there a time perspective bias you lean towards, and how do you feel about your scores? How can you shift your time perspective so that it becomes more balanced? Write your thoughts below.

> **Sample Strategies to Strengthen Each Time Perspective**
>
> **Past-positive time perspective:** reexperience past happiness
>
> **Present-pleasure time perspective:** immerse yourself in happiness and pleasure in the present
>
> **Future time perspective:** plan to be happy in future and derive pleasure from expectation of future happiness.

Now that you know your time perspective, which strategies can you use in Table 11.2 to strengthen a time perspective that you are perhaps not utilising so much? My experience of coaching dental professionals has highlighted that many of us struggle with prioritising the present orientation.

Table 11.2 Time perspective strengthening strategies.

Time perspective	Strategies to strengthen this time perspective
Future-orientated	• Set goals for the future, for example, today, tomorrow, and within the next month. • Create a vision board. • Chart your progress towards your goal. • Practice mental visualisation. • Make to-do lists, ranking most important to least. • Work towards long-term bigger rewards instead settling for short-term quick ones.
Present-orientated	• Ground yourself using mindfulness. • Try physical exercise that focuses on breathwork, for example, pilates or yoga. • Get engrossed in a book. • Go outside for a nature hike. • Practice sensual pleasures, for example, long shower, aromatherapy. • Play with your children. • Play with pets. • Plan for periods of spontaneity, for example, set aside a weekend day and make no plans for it.
Past-positive-orientated	• Send a gratitude letter to a loved one. • Create a gratitude jar, with your gratitude points for the day, and reread them occasionally. • Make a travel scrapbook. • Call an old friend and reminisce about your shared past. • Place pictures of happy memories around home.

The Optimal Time Perspective

A balanced time orientation, rather than having a bias towards one particular time perspective, helps us to shift our attention easily between past, present, and future and adapt our mindset to any situation. The benefits are enormous: we develop a greater work–life balance as well as greater psychological and physical well-being. What does this look like? Zimbardo's extensive research proposes an optimal time perspective, summarised in Table 11.3.

Table 11.3   Optimal time perspective levels.

Optimal time perspective	Levels
Past-positive	High
Present-pleasure	Moderate (but selected, self-rewarding, and not impulsive)
Future	Moderately high
Past-negative	Low
Past-fatalistic	Low

Time Perspective and Paths to Happiness

A biased time perspective can close potential doors to our happiness. Many of us as dental professionals may have a bias towards future orientation, which leads us to cultivate strategies to develop conscientiousness to study, grit, and set life goals. The journey may mean sacrificing our own well-being, hobbies, family, and so forth to get there. A balanced time perspective provides mental flexibility and opens all paths to happiness.

We can utilise time to increase our levels of positive emotions. Figure 11.1 combines the work of Zimbardo with Sonja Lyubomirsky's evidence-based happiness strategies (Lyubomirsky 2007; see Chapter 2).

HAPPINESS
GYM

Zambardo and Sonja Lyobomirsky's evidenced based happiness strategies

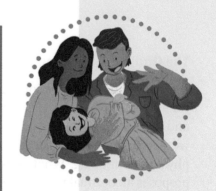

PRESENT

- Savour life's joys
- Increase flow experiences
- Practise acts of kindness
- Mindfulness
- Nuture relationships

POSITIVE PAST

- Gratitude
- Avoid over thinking or rumination
- Learn to forgive

FUTURE

- Taking care of your body
- Set and pursue life goals
- Develop coping strategies

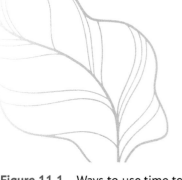

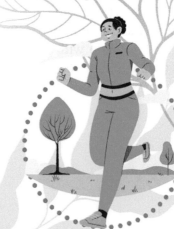

Figure 11.1 Ways to use time to increase levels of positive emotions. Lasse Kristensen / Adobe Stock.

Developing An Optimistic Future
Using Best Possible Self

Imagine your life in the future – for example, five years from now. Imagine that everything has gone as well as it possibly could and you've realised all your dreams. Describe how you are feeling, the steps you took to achieve your goals, the strengths you used, and how you overcame any obstacles on the way. Write about this below, noting all the small details. Adapted from Meevissen et al. 2011.

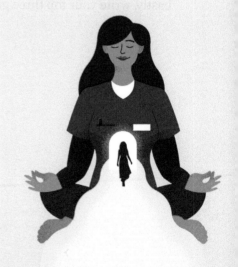

Time for Change

The key message from the research on time is the importance of carving personalised moments in our day over an emphasis on filling our days to the brim. It takes time for change. Anticipate some setbacks. Prioritise learning to relax and, as always, be self-compassionate during this process.

Tips To Personalise Your Time

- Identify what you enjoy and what matters to you the most. Then amplify!
- Practise mindfulness. Being present allows us to slow down, feel engaged with our life, and be witness to the small pleasures of our every day.
- Introduce psychological 'white space' – time during the day where you get to daydream and zone, rather than packing your days to the brim.
- Zoom out and look for links between your time use and your values. Are your activities aligned with your values?
- Draw on your strengths – use these more often in your day to boost your well-being.

Are you interested in applying positive psychology to plan your best day? Try the *My Daily Positive Planner* worksheet. Start with thinking your mission possible for the day, your most important tasks, and which action points you need to take. Consider your top values and character strengths you can employ next to help you achieve your mission. Consider rewards that can add pleasure to your day. Write down positive statements that can help you with your tasks. Lastly, write your top three gratitude points in the evening.

My Daily
Positive Planner

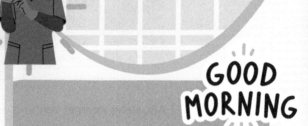

My Positive Mantras:

Values & Strengths I
want to use today:

GOOD MORNING

My Mission Possibles:

My Top 3 Wins:

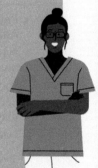

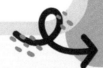

Well-Being, Play, and Dentistry

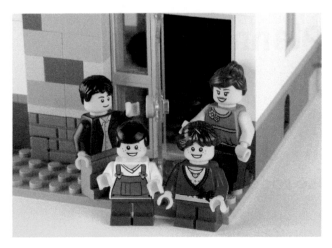

ABC News Internet Ventures.

When was the last time you played? As busy professionals we could really benefit from giving ourselves permission to play! There are many benefits of play as adults. In this section, we explore what play is, the research findings, especially on how play enriches our well-being, and how we can apply this exciting research to our lives.

Play can be defined as 'an activity that is carried out for the purpose of amusement and fun, that is approached with an enthusiastic and in the moment attitude' (Van Vleet and Feeney 2015). Playfulness is also a personality trait, with some of us having a higher tendency to engage in play.

Types of play	Benefits of play for dental professionals
• Physical play: active exercise, running, climbing • Symbolic play: playing with language, imagery/drawing, music, numbers • Socio-dramatic play: acting out narratives, characters, situations, playing with identities, and stories • Games with rules: board games	• Increases our resilience, reduces stress, and enhances ability to cope with adversities • Buffers against imposter syndrome thoughts • Increases creativity and ability to think 'outside the box' • Enhances our relationships with patients, colleagues, and at home • Increases our physical fitness, life satisfaction, hope, emotional and intellectual strengths (Proyer and Ruch 2011)

The Broaden-and-Build Theory may explain why play is so beneficial to adults. Play enhances our levels of positive emotions, broadens our thinking, and helps us to build psychosocial resources and strengths, including resilience. This in turn may cause an upwards spiral of further positive emotions. Michele Tugade and Barbara Fredrickson's research highlighted that resilient people use positive emotions to bounce back from negative experiences, finding meaning in adversities and speeding cardiovascular recovery from negative arousal (Tugade and Fredrickson 2004, 2007). Resilient people use positive emotions to build resilience and cope with stressful events.

Table 11.4 summarises the research findings on the benefits of play in adults.

Table 11.4   Benefits of play in adults.

Well-being measure	Research findings
Coping and resilience	• In university students, playful individuals report lower perceived stress and make more use of active, adaptive, and less avoidant, negative coping strategies (Magnuson and Barnett 2013). • Individuals high in playfulness are less prone to experiencing personal stress and more likely to engage in leisure activities to manage stress (Staempfli 2007).
Well-being and happiness	• Playfulness positively associated with physical fitness, life satisfaction, active lifestyles, and well-being (Proyer 2013). • Associated with humour and happiness in Chinese adults (Yue et al. 2016).
Creativity	• Associated with creativity (Proyer and Ruch 2011).
Relationships at work and dating	• Playfulness supports innovative work performance (Glynn and Webster 1992). • Associated with teamwork (Proyer and Ruch 2011). • Playfulness is a preferred trait in potential partners (Proyer and Wagner 2015).
Positive psychological functioning and ageing	• Playfulness in older adults associated with well-being, cognitive-emotional functioning, and healthy ageing (Yarnal and Qian 2011). • Positively associated with agreeableness, higher internally motivated goals, and better academic performance (Proyer 2011, 2012)

Think About It

Inviting More Play

Which play activities can you schedule in your day? Use the illustrations below for some suggestions and write these down:

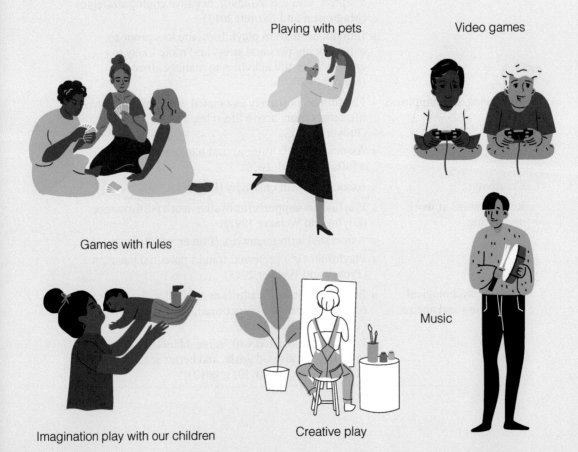

Playing with pets

Video games

Games with rules

Music

Imagination play with our children

Creative play

Design Your Own Intervention

Try this play intervention: Create a 'play jar' by adding your play activities into a jar and picking one a day for the next week. Notice how this intervention impacts your well-being.

Digital Well-Being

Around 40% of the world's population (that is, around three billion people) use social media and spend an average of two hours daily liking, commenting, sharing, and updating their virtual platforms. Within dentistry, social media is widely used in business as a powerful platform for associates to practice owners to offer exposure on a level that would not have been possible a few decades ago. With the possibility to tap into virtual communities and reduce distances through connecting with people from around the globe, our phones have the beautiful capacity to connect us and at the same time present us with so many challenges when it comes to managing our time and well-being.

Despite social media being considered a popular leisure activity around the world, prolonged social media use has many profound impacts on our psychological well-being. Table 11.5 summarises the psychological fallout of prolonged social media use and the mechanisms in how they work to undercut our well-being.

Table 11.5 The risks of social media.

Risk of excessive social media use/ addiction	Mechanism and research
Reduced self-esteem	• Opinions of other people, either friends or public, and the feedback from them have a very strong effect on our self-esteem. • We are wired to socially connect, so what other people think of us matters. • Dentistry is a very visual profession, with images of our clinical work, from composite bonding to implant placement, being featured on social media. Engaging in upwards social comparison (evaluations based on skill, popularity – that is, number of likes – engagement, wealth accumulation, beauty, awards, and so on) can make us feel like we are not 'good enough' and foster negative evaluations of ourselves. This results in reduced self-esteem (Lockwood and Kunda 1997). • One hour spent on Facebook daily results in a decrease in the self-esteem score of an individual (Jan et al. 2017). • Researchers at Penn State University suggested that seeing other people's selfies lowered self-esteem (Wang et al. 2017). The authors suggested this may be because users compare themselves to photos of people looking their happiest. Frequent selfie viewing led to decreased life satisfaction, with the need for popularity moderating the relationship between selfie viewing and self-esteem and life satisfaction.
Increased stress	• Women reported higher stress levels than men in one study of 1800 participants (Hampton et al. 2015). The average adult in their sample knew people who had experienced 5 of the 12 major life events, for example, a robbery to engagements, divorce to accidents. Twitter was found to be a 'significant contributor' to stress because it highlighted awareness of other people's stress.
Lower mood	• Researchers in Austria reported use of Facebook for 20 minutes resulted in lower moods in participants. Authors suggested this was due to participants feeling like this time was a waste of their time (Sagioglou and Greitemeyer 2014). The authors commented on a cause for excessive Facebook usage: people commit a forecasting error by expecting to feel better after Facebook use.
Reduced well-being	• Social media has a more negative effect on the well-being of those who are more socially isolated.

Table 11.5 (Continued)

Risk of excessive social media use/addiction	Mechanism and research
Sleep disturbances	• One large study of 1700 18- to 30-year-olds on their social media and sleeping habits reported an association with sleep disturbances (Levenson et al. 2016). The authors suggested that blue light had a part to play. The physiological arousal before sleep, and the bright lights of our phones, can delay our circadian rhythms. Obsessive checking of social media as opposed to time spent on it was the highest predictor of disturbed sleep.
Relationships	• Excessive use linked with relationship problems. • The presence of a phone can interfere with our face-to-face interactions. • In a small study, 34 pairs of strangers had a 10-minute conversation about an interesting event that had happened to them recently (Przybylski and Weinstein 2013). Half had a mobile phone on the top of their table, whereas the other half had a notebook. Those with a phone on the table reported less meaningful conversations and reduced closeness with their partner. The authors suggested this may be due to mobile phones triggering automatic negative thoughts about wider social networks, which has the effect of crowding out face-to-face conversations.
Addiction	• Social media addiction is considered by some researchers to be a mental health problem that 'may' require professional treatment (Kuss and Griffiths 2011). • The authors reviewed 43 studies, reporting excessive usage was linked to worse academic achievement and reduced participation in offline communities. The people most at risk could be those dependent on alcohol, those who are highly extroverted, and those who use social media to compensate for fewer ties in real life.
Anxiety	• Researchers have studied the relationship between anxiety and social media usage by examining feelings of restlessness and worry and trouble sleeping and concentrating. • One study reported a significant association between the number of social media platforms and anxiety and depression. The participants who used seven or more social media platforms were more than 3 times as likely as people using 0–2 platforms to have high levels of general anxiety symptoms (Primack et al. 2017). Authors suggested reasons may include cyber-bullying, having a distorted view of other people's lives, and feeling like time spent on social media is a waste.
Depression	• Two studies involving more than 700 students found that depressive symptoms were greater among those who reported having more negative interactions online (Davila et al. 2012).

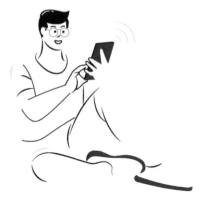

As with all technology, we need to be mindful about interacting with it intentionally. Fortunately, there are a number of positive steps we can take to enhance our mental well-being whilst using social media. Here are some suggestions based on positive psychology, mindfulness, and cognitive-behavioural therapy. As with all mind tools, experiment with the strategies to work out which work best for you.

- *Start your day mindfully and stop those 'stress hits' piling up.*
  Avoid checking in with social media the moment you wake. Our brains have evolved to be highly attuned to danger – it used to be the sabre-toothed tiger, but now any negative news on social media is seen as a threat.

- *Increase self-awareness of your social media triggers and behaviours.*
  Ensure you check in and identify which posts are feeding your brain positive emotion versus the negatives.

- *Increase your levels of positive emotions.*
  Curate a feed that is positive and uplifting by following accounts that raise your levels of joy, optimism, humour, and a zest for learning.

- *Encourage a positive mindset by minimising the impact of negative thoughts using thinking judo.*
  Upwards social comparison with others may lead to overcritical, catastrophising thoughts centred on being 'good enough'. This cycle of negative thoughts underpins anxiety and depression. Dentistry is also a visual results-focused profession, which may magnify this negativity. Minimise time spent in thinking traps by actively practising the 3Cs (as described in Chapter 8):

- **Catch** a negative thought.
- **Check** it – is this thought helping me or hindering me?
- **Change** it using three thinking strategies:

1) Examine the evidence ('This is not true because. . .')
2) Reframe ('A more helpful way to think about this. . .') or
3) Plan ('If X happens, I will do this. . .').

Actively practising the above, in real time, rewires your brain to become resilient. Our brains have amazing neuroplasticity – and can create new neural pathways for resilience each time they are exercised.

- *Limit the time spent on social media.*
  Use tracking apps and schedule pockets of the day or use scheduling apps that automatically post to help you reduce time spent online.

- *Practise self-awareness and self-compassion.*
  If you catch yourself unnecessarily scrolling for a long period, ask yourself: 'Is this helping or hindering me?', 'How am I feeling?', 'How is my body feeling?', 'What do I really need in this moment?'. As humans wired for social connectedness, we may be feeling lonely. Consider alternative activities that you can do rather than aimlessly reaching for your phone. Write a list of options and keep these to hand. Whenever you have a spare couple of minutes, try one of these activities instead of social media.

- *Use your most underrated social media superpower – the power of muting.*
  Turn off notifications. Constant alerts will tire and stress the brain. If switching off alerts is not possible, create boundaries that help you unplug during parts of the day.

- *Be kind to yourself by avoiding engagement with trolls.*
  Delete the comment and use the 3Cs above if you feel triggered.

- *Take a digital detox two hours before bed.*
  Turn your phone to airplane mode. Enjoy your downtime and a good night's sleep.

The *Digital Well-being Checklist* summarises the digital well-being tips discussed in this section. Use these as prompts to help you establish a new relationship with your tech usage.

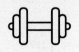

Digital Well-being Checklist

- ✔ I start my day mindfully, avoiding social media first thing
- ✔ I increase my awareness of my social comparison triggers
- ✔ I increase my positive emotions by curating a positive feed
- ✔ I limit time spent of social media using apps
- ✔ I turn off notifications
- ✔ I post content that's meaningful to me
- ✔ When I catch negative self talk after seeing a past I soothe myself with self-compassion
- ✔ I unfollow toxic accounts & avoid engaging trolls
- ✔ I celebrate others wins on social media
- ✔ I practise digital detox 1 hour before bed

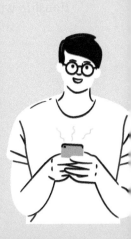

Prioritising Digital Well-being

1. Which social media apps/tech do you use most often? How does your use impact your time and well-being?

2. If you had extra time in your day, which activities would you love to do more of that bring you pleasure? Write this list below to give you ideas for activities you can do instead of reaching for your phone. How can you reduce your social media/tech use to make time for the activities listed?

Activities I want to do more of	Ways I can reduce my tech use?

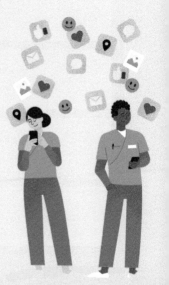

Caring Technology

One of the greatest missions of positive psychology is to encourage global flourishing. The potential of caring technology and smartphone-based well-being interventions may play a vital role. Research into well-being apps supports that the viability of smartphone-based interventions may significantly enhance our wellness. As with all interventions, acknowledging the role of person–activity fit is key. Table 11.6 summarises how different types of apps can benefit us in different ways.

Table 11.6 The benefits of apps.

Type of app	Benefits
Health tracker app	• Increases our self-knowledge and awareness (Lupton 2017) – people look to these devices to see how they are feeling. • People feel happy when the numbers look good, but they feel unsettled and nervous when the numbers look bad (Sumartojo et al. 2016). • Your personality traits impact how you feel and how you use health tracker apps – for example, harmonious positive passion for physical exercise predicts positive benefits from fitness apps and is negatively associated with burnout. An obsessive negative passion is predicted by increases of burnout (Whelan and Clohessy 2021).
Psychological well-being app	• Bakker and Rickard (2018) researched MoodPrism, an emotional well-being app, and discovered that engagement predicted decrease in depression and anxiety and increase in well-being mediated by an increase in emotional self-awareness. • Clarke and Draper (2020) studied Calm, a mindfulness app, and discovered that daily and intermittent use increased trait mindfulness, self-efficacy, and well-being. However, qualitive data revealed that some participants had some very negative experiences. Take home message: doesn't work for everyone, and you need to mindful of your personal experience. • McEwan et al. (2019) looked at a well-being app for connecting with urban nature. Participants were guided to notice the good things about urban nature or built spaces. The authors discovered significant, sustained increase in well-being at one-month follow-up for both clinical and non-clinical participants. The authors suggested this may be due to increases in nature connectedness and increases in positive emotions.

Summary

- How we view time impacts our behaviours.
- Zimbardo identified five different ways we spend thinking about time.
- Optimal time perspective is high in past-positive, moderate in present-pleasure and future, low in past-negative and past-fatalistic.
- Increase time affluence through personalising your time by identifying what you enjoy, be mindful, schedule psychological white space, and draw on values and strengths.
- Prioritising play is good for us! We can reap the well-being benefits of play by doing more 'play' activities, such as board games, sports games, playing with Lego, and colouring.
- Increase your digital well-being by curating a positive feed, catch negative thoughts, limit your time on social media, mute notifications, increase self-awareness of social media triggers, and digital detox two hours before bedtime.

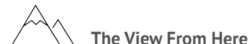 **The View From Here**

My days used to be filled to the brim. Which makes a lot of sense, as I work as a dentist, a teacher, and a coach and I write. I also create well-being products. The appeal of being as productive as I can meant that prioritising downtime and rest always felt like such a struggle. But this also resulted in me feeling more like I was drowning in the sea of endless tasks. I realised that my resilience levels were quickly diminishing, and this led me to reach out to my own coach, who laid it on thick. I was on the road to burnout again and needed to do a whole lot less if I wanted to be happier and healthier. This led me on the journey to start integrating positive psychology lessons to my life, the first one being working on my relationship with time. We all have the power to examine our schedules, work out what matters the most, and take small steps in shifting to a work–life harmony that nourishes us. It will look different for all of us. And our time certainly doesn't need to be equally divided; in fact, that isn't possible. However, we can make strides in personalising our time better, curating a day that incorporates rest, pleasure, curiosity, and meaning. What does that look like for you?

References

Bakker, D. and Rickard, N. (2018). Engagement in mobile phone app for self-monitoring of emotional wellbeing predicts changes in mental health: MoodPrism. *Journal of Affective Disorders* 227: 432–442.

Clarke, J. and Draper, S. (2020). Intermittent mindfulness practice can be beneficial, and daily practice can be harmful. An in depth, mixed methods study of the 'Calm' app's (mostly positive) effects. *Internet Interventions* 19: 100293. ISSN: 2214-7829.

Davila, J., Hershenberg, R., Feinstein, B.A. et al. (2012). Frequency and quality of social networking among young adults: associations with depressive symptoms, rumination, and corumination. *Psychology of Popular Media Culture* 1 (2): 72–86.

Glynn, M.A. and Webster, J. (1992). The adult playfulness scale: an initial assessment. *Psychological Reports* 71 (1): 83–103.

Hampton, K., Rainie, L., Lu, W. et al. (2015). Social media and the cost of caring. Pew Research Center. https://www.pewresearch.org/internet/2015/01/15/social-media-and-stress/

Hodgkinson, T. (2005). *How to Be Idle*. New York: Harper Collins Publishers.

Holman, E.A. and Zimbardo, P.G. (2009). The social language of time: the time perspective–social network connection. *Basic and Applied Social Psychology* 31 (2): 136–147.

Jan, M., Soomro, S., and Ahmad, N. (2017). Impact of social media on self-esteem. *European Scientific Journal* 13 (23): 329–341.

Kuss, D.J. and Griffiths, M.D. (2011). Online social networking and addiction – a review of the psychological literature. *International Journal of Environmental Research and Public Health* 8 (9): 3528–3552.

Levenson, J.C., Shensa, A., Sidani, J.E. et al. (2016). The association between social media use and sleep disturbance among young adults. *Preventive Medicine* 85: 36–41.

Lockwood, P. and Kunda, Z. (1997). Superstars and me: predicting the impact of role models on the self. *Journal of Personality and Social Psychology* 73: 91–103.

Lupton, D. (2017). Self-tracking, health and medicine. *Health Sociology Review* 26: 1–5. https://doi.org/10.1080/14461242.2016.1228149.

Lyubomirsky, S. (2007). *The How of Happiness: A Scientific Approach to Getting the Life You Want*. Penguin Press.

Magnuson, C. and Barnett, L. (2013). The playful advantage: how playfulness enhances coping with stress. *Leisure Sciences* 35 (2): 129–144.

McEwan, K., Richardson, M., Sheffield, D. et al. (2019). A smartphone app for improving mental health through connecting with urban nature. *International Journal of Environmental Research and Public Health* 16 (18): 3373.

Meevissen, Y.M.C., Peters, M.L., and Alberts, H.J.E.M. (2011). Become more optimistic by imagining a best possible self: effects of a two week intervention. *Journal of Behaviour Therapy and Experimental Psychiatry* 42: 371–378.

Mello, Z.R. and Worrell, F.C. (2006). The relationship of time perspective to age, gender, and academic achievement among academically talented adolescents. *Journal for the Education of the Gifted* 29 (3): 271–289.

Primack, B., Shensa, A., Escobar-Viera, C. et al. (2017). Use of multiple social media platforms and symptoms of depression and anxiety: a nationally-representative study among U.S. young adults. *Computers in Human Behavior* 69: 1–9.

Proyer, R. (2011). Being playful and smart? The relations of adult playfulness with psychometric and self-estimated intelligence and academic performance. *Learning and Individual Differences* 21: 463–467. https://doi.org/10.1016/j.lindif.2011.02.003.

Proyer, R. (2012). Examining playfulness in adults: testing its correlates with personality, positive psychological functioning, goal aspirations, and multi-methodically assessed ingenuity. *Psychological Test and Assessment Modeling* 54: https://doi.org/10.5167/uzh-63532.

Proyer, R. (2013). The well-being of playful adults: adult playfulness, subjective well-being, physical well-being, and the pursuit of enjoyable activities. *European Journal of Humour Research* 1: 84–98. https://doi.org/10.5167/uzh-78008.

Proyer, René & Ruch, Willibald. (2011). The virtuousness of adult playfulness: the relation of playfulness with strengths of character. *Psychology of Well-Being: Theory, Research and Practice*1, 4.

Proyer, R. and Wagner, L. (2015). Playfulness in adults revisited: the signal theory in German speakers. *American Journal of Play* 7: 201–227. https://doi.org/10.5167/uzh-110043.

Przybylski, A.K. and Weinstein, N. (2013). Can you connect with me now? How the presence of mobile communication technology influences face-to-face conversation quality. *Journal of Social and Personal Relationships* 30 (3): 237–246.

Sagioglou, C. and Greitemeyer, T. (2014). Facebook's emotional consequences: why Facebook causes a decrease in mood and why people still use it. *Computers in Human Behavior* 35: 359–363.

Staempfli, M. (2007). Adolescent playfulness, stress perception, coping and well being. *Journal of Leisure Research* 39: 393–412.

Sumartojo, S., Pink, S., and Lupton, D. (2016). The affective intensities of datafied space. *Emotion, Space and Society* 21: 33–40.

Tugade, M.M. and Fredrickson, B.L. (2004). Resilient individuals use positive emotions to bounce back from negative emotional experiences. *Journal of Personality and Social Psychology* 86 (2): 320–333.

Tugade, M.M. and Fredrickson, B.L. (2007). Regulation of positive emotions: emotion regulation strategies that promote resilience. *Journal of Happiness Studies: An Interdisciplinary Forum on Subjective Well-Being* 8 (3): 311–333.

Van Vleet, M. and Feeney, B.C. (2015). Young at heart: a perspective for advancing research on play in adulthood. *Perspectives on Psychological Science* 10 (5): 639–645.

Wang, R., Yang, F., and Haigh, M.M. (2017). Let me take a selfie: exploring the psychological effects of posting and viewing selfies and groupies on social media. *Telematics and Informatics* 34 (4): 274–283.

Whelan, E. and Clohessy, T. (2021). *How the social dimension of fitness apps can enhance and undermine wellbeing: a dual model of passion perspective*, vol. 34, 68–92. Information Technology and People.

Yarnal, C. and Qian, X. (2011). Older-adult playfulness: an innovative construct and measurement for healthy aging research. *American Journal of Play* 4: 52–79.

Yue, X.D., Leung, C.-L., and Hiranandani, N.A. (2016). Adult playfulness, humor styles, and subjective happiness. *Psychological Reports* 119 (3): 630–640.

Zimbardo, P.G. and Boyd, J. (2008). *The Time Paradox: The New Psychology of Time that Will Change Your Life*. Atria Books.

12

Designing Habits That Stick

CHAPTER OVERVIEW

- Understanding motivation
- Increasing self-confidence
- Behaviour change
- Goal setting
- Pro tips for designing habits that stick.

Now that we know more about well-being tools, the next step to increasing our wellness is to understand how we can design habits that stick. Every aspect of our lives is built on habits, from our weekly gym sessions to brushing our teeth twice a day. All of us will be very familiar with the obstacles to integrating positive habits in our lives. Laziness, distraction, and forgetfulness are three common hindrances. With many of the habits discussed in this book, from practising gratitude and mindfulness to self-compassion, gratification and results are delayed. This means that instead of relying on willpower, we need to intelligently design ways we can build positive habits that stick. In this chapter, we explore how to do this, delving into motivation, the creation of habits, and a new way to design habits.

Motivation

The most common myth around behaviour change is that we need more motivation. If we had more motivation, we would be able to consistently and easily integrate new habits. The flaw with this thinking is that many of us do indeed know of the benefits of the new behaviour we are trying to implement, and we may also know the risks of not successfully integrating the habits. Whilst motivation can help us in the short term, psychologists highlight that it is not the crucial fuel in keeping us committed to long-term behaviour change. There are other factors at play: namely our self-confidence, known as self-efficacy, our

Resilience and Well-being for Dental Professionals, First Edition. Mahrukh Khwaja.
© 2023 John Wiley & Sons Ltd. Published 2023 by John Wiley & Sons Ltd.
Companion website: www.wiley.com/go/khwaja-resilience-dentistry

values, and, if this behaviour integrates with them, the design of the behaviour change and our mindset.

To begin with, let's break down the science of motivation.

1) Motivation is energy for action.

2) It is not the amount of motivation that is key, more the type of motivation.

3) Psychologists Edward Deci and Richard Ryan highlighted two types of motivation in their Self-Determination Theory (Deci and Ryan 1985, 2000). For the purposes of illustrating the two types in a more engaging way, I will use metaphors. One type of motivation is a lot like *junk food* (extrinsic motivation): it tastes good but does not offer us great nutritional value. This is where the drive to do the habit is based on external forces, such as money, acclaim, the threat of punishment, or the promise of reward. We can think of this type of motivation as a habit that we do because we *have* to. The second type of motivation can be thought of as *high-quality healthy food* (intrinsic motivation): it nourishes our body both mentally and physically. This is a type of motivation where the drive to do the task is more for inherent enjoyment and satisfaction for the action itself. We *want* to do it.

4) We can design all our goals and create habits that stick by increasing our 'high quality' motivation. To create conditions to increase our 'quality' motivation, we need to increase all our needs for motivation; that is, choice (having options and the choice to decide for ourself), competence (having the right skills for the task), and connection (social connection with others).

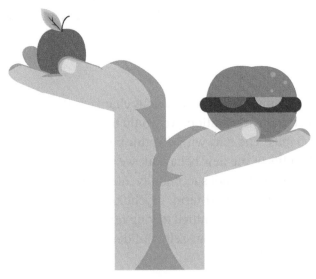

High quality motivation (intrinsic motivation) vs Low quality motivation (extrinsic motivation)

beats_ / Adobe Stock.

Increasing 'Quality' Motivation

Reflect on a recent goal that you have been trying to implement. What is the driver for the goal? Is it for external reasons or because you inherently enjoy or find the goal meaningful? How can you frame the goal in a way that sits with your values and increases your 'quality' motivation?

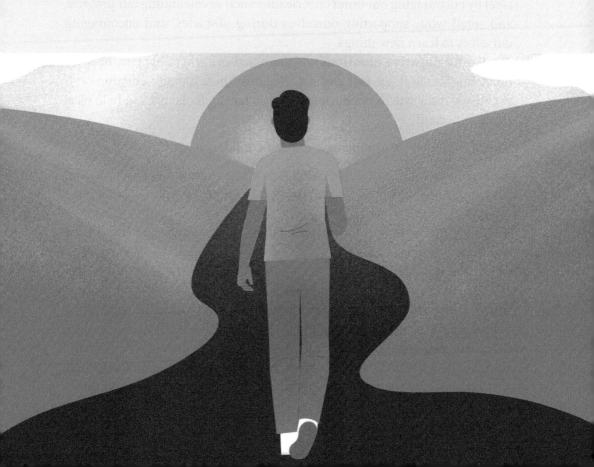

Tapping into Self-Confidence

Self-confidence, known as self-efficacy, is an important psychological construct describing our belief in our ability to get a specific task done. Unsurprisingly, our self-confidence level impacts our choices, goal setting, effort, and persistence. We are much more likely to achieve difficult goals and try again after rejections if we have higher levels of self-confidence.

We have all felt our confidence waver or felt anxious about our ability to overcome a problem we face. Sometimes goals can be daunting and difficult – this is where self-efficacy matters the most. Albert Bandura describes four routes to increasing our self confidence in his Self-Efficacy Theory of Motivation (Bandura 1977):

1) **Previous positive experiences:** Reflecting on past experiences where we did well helps to remind us that we can succeed and feel more confident.
2) **Role modelling:** Seeing others succeed is a powerful way to increase our belief that we can also succeed.
3) **Words of encouragement:** When we were children, words of encouragement came from our primary caregivers. As an adult, we can tap into this facet by encouraging our inner cheerleader, such as celebrating our progress and small wins, supporting ourselves during obstacles, and encouraging ourselves to learn new things.
4) **Managing negative emotions:** As discussed in earlier chapters, how we think impacts how we feel and act. Negative thoughts and emotions can negatively influence our behaviours, and so having tools that can help us is really important.

Using this model, we can increase our self-confidence by:

- **Mastering tasks:** For example, public speaking improvement by attending speaking groups, such as Toastmasters. This increases our positive past experiences.
- **Modelling behaviour:** Find role models to observe and gain inspiration from seeing others succeed.
- **Social persuasion:** Finding mentors or coaches to help build our self-confidence.
- **Improve emotional regulation:** This can be done through using tools, such as mindfulness, self-compassion, and cognitive-behavioural therapy (CBT). We can also interpret our physiological response differently; for example, the adrenaline and anxiety from public speaking can be reframed as excitement and gratitude that you're alert and ready to deliver your talk

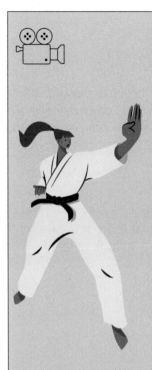

Learning From Movies

A Case Study: Karate Kid

The *Karate Kid* tells the story of a teenager, Daniel, who moves to Southern California with his mother. He quickly finds himself the target of bullies who study karate at a training centre, Cobra Kai. Luckily, Daniel befriends Mr. Miyagi, a former martial arts master who trains him in a more compassionate form of karate and prepares him to compete against his bullies. Aside from being a classic coming-of-age story, *Karate Kid* charts the journey of Daniel to self-confidence as described by Bandura: Mr. Miyagi becomes an excellent role model for Daniel, he nurtures words of encouragement and support in the form of lessons, such as the famous 'wax on and wax off' scene, and he helps Daniel work through negative emotions through channelling his anger into patience, persistence, and faith.

Addressing Negative Thoughts

Using the cognitive reappraisal tool, we can reframe our negative thoughts whilst we are working our way to achieve our goals. Start by writing down any negative thoughts that pop up in your mind around a goal you want to achieve. Write this down in the first column. Next, write down the evidence against this thought. In the final column, note a more helpful way of seeing this.

Negative thought	Evidence against this thought	A more helpful way to look at this is...

Understanding Behaviour Change

Armed with your knowledge of motivation, self-confidence, and the role of mindset, understanding the steps in behaviour change is our next step. The Transtheoretical Model of Change (Figure 12.1; Prochaska and DiClemente 1983) describes the six stages in creating behaviour change.

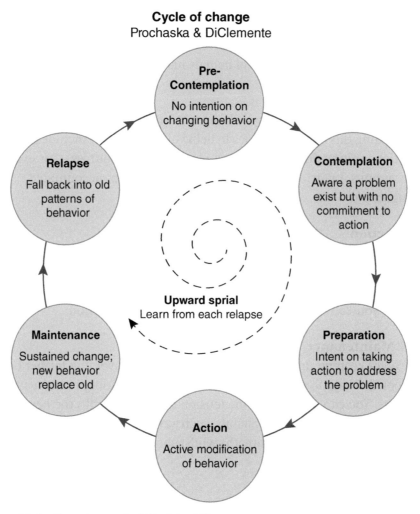

Figure 12.1   Transtheoretical Model of Change.

Stage 1: Precontemplation

This is the earliest stage and describes when we are not even considering a change. We feel that the behaviour isn't a problem. We can begin the process of moving through the stages of change by reflecting on the risks of this behaviour.

Stage 2: Contemplation

This stage can last months to even years. During this stage, individuals become increasingly aware of the benefits of making a change, but the costs of that change stand out more. This creates a sense of conflict about changing. We can move from this stage by asking ourselves why we want to change, what our obstacles are, and things that could help us make the change.

Stage 3: Preparation

In this stage we are making small changes to prepare for a larger life change, such as reading this book! Strategies to help you in this stage include gathering information, writing down goals and a plan, finding resources – for example, support groups or friends that can help you keep accountable – and encouragement.

Stage 4: Action

During this stage, individuals take action to fulfil their goals. Taking time to review your motivation for the behaviour, resources, progress, and support is important in helping maintain positive movement towards behaviour change. Rewarding yourself can also help you to continue taking action.

Stage 5: Maintenance

This involves keeping up with the new behaviour and avoiding former behaviours. Look for ways to avoid temptation through scheduling in the new habit in fun ways. You can also reduce the tension to continue with the new behaviour by piggybacking off existing habits, such as mindfully eating the first three bites of lunch or mindful deep breaths whilst showering. Remember to reward yourself for avoiding relapses.

Stage 6: Relapse

With all behaviour changes, relapses are common. In fact, some studies report as high as three times around the model before a new behaviour sticks. If you falter, try self-compassion and remind yourself that this relapse is common and part of the process of making a change. Reflect on the triggers to relapse and consider how you can avoid these in the future. Reaffirm your goal and your commitment to making change.

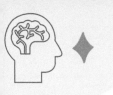

Think About It

Stages of Change

Which behaviours have you been recently thinking about integrating? Which stage are you on the model described above? Have you relapsed? What are the barriers to success for you? How can you minimise these?

Mindset and Behaviour Change

A growth mindset during behaviour change is necessary in being able to navigate setbacks and encourage ourselves to continue to engage with behaviour change. As discussed in Chapter 8, Carol Dweck's research unearths the power of mindset. If we approach our goals with a growth rather than fixed mindset, we can motivate ourselves to reach professional and personal goals successfully. We can teach ourselves to thrive on challenge, rather than be reduced by it. We can move towards a growth mindset through believing that we can learn new things, reframing relapses as stepping stones to successfully implementing our new behaviour, and praising our progress. It's certainly not always easy, but growing one's mindset and changing the way we think about learning can help to fulfil our highest potential.

Goal-Setting 101

When done correctly, goal setting can be a powerful tool for productivity and making habits that stick. Locke's Goal-Setting Theory (Locke 1968; Locke and Latham 1990) identifies five characteristics of setting goals successfully; clarity, challenge, commitment, feedback, and task complexity:

Clarity: To be motivating, goals need to be clear. We can do this by setting SMART goals, understand how we will hit our goal, and use a metric to track progress.

Challenge: Goals need to hit the sweet spot between challenging and not overchallenging you. We can do this by setting realistic goals.

Commitment: You need to be committed to achieving the goal. We can gain commitment through using visualisation techniques, where we imagine achieving our goals, and rewarding ourselves as we make progress with our goal.

Feedback: Receiving feedback is effective in goal setting and helps us track our progress.

Task complexity: Good goal setting involves breaking down goals into sub-goals, ensuring goals are not too complicated. This helps us to avoid feeling overwhelmed.

Developing Grit

Grit is also closely connected with goal setting. In psychology, grit is a positive trait focused on an individual's perseverance of effort with passion for a specific long-term goal. Research by professor of psychology Angela Duckworth and colleagues describes grit as the secret sauce when it comes to our success, and it is considered a more influential predictor of achievement than our IQ (Duckworth 2006). Duckworth speculates that grit may be particularly important to especially challenging goals, where the temptation to give up is high, whereas self-discipline is more key for more moderate tasks that are highly structured. If you're upskilling in dentistry, running a practice, or starting a big project, grit is crucial in getting you there.

Here are four ways we can increase our levels of grit:

1) **Discover what you are passionate about** by reflecting on what really interests you.
2) **Pay focused attention** to your goal. Make a plan, set small subgoals, and take small steps.
3) **Create a sense of purpose,** and this will help you to maintain grit, especially during challenging times.
4) **Cultivate a growth mindset:** This involves cultivating self-compassion, speaking to ourselves in a kinder way, reminding ourselves of our progress over perfection, and reframing failure as stepping stones to success.

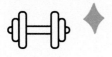

Goal Mapping

6. How can you **reward** yourself for making progress with your goal?

5. How can you track your **progress**?

4. How can you obtain **feedback** regarding the goal?

3. If things don't go according to plan, what can you **try**?

2. What are the **small steps** needed in order to achieve this goal?

1. Write down a **goal** that you want to implement in the next 6 months.

GROW Model

Goal	Reality	Options	Will
What do you want?	Where are you now?	What could you do?	What will you do?

The GROW model is a framework for goal setting and problem solving, developed in the UK by Sir John Whitmore and colleagues in the late 1980s. Although it is used most extensively in corporate coaching, the GROW model can help us work through designing our goals.

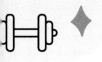

Goal Setting Using GROW

1. **Goal:** What would you like to work on? What are the benefits for you in achieving this goal? When will you do this?

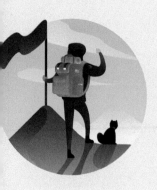

2. **Reality:** What will it be like if you achieve your goal? What will you see/hear/feel?

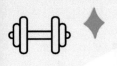

Goal Setting Using GROW

3. What action have you taken so far? What is getting in the way?

4. **Options:** What options do you have for achieving your goal? What are the pros and cons for each option? Which option will you try first?

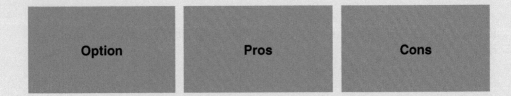

Option	Pros	Cons

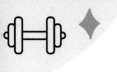

Option	Pros	Cons

5. **Will**: When will you start each action? What support can you ask for to help you? How committed are you, on a scale of 0–10, to taking these actions? If not a 10, what would make it a 10?

Pro Tips to Designing Habits That Stick

In this chapter, we discussed how creating a new behaviour takes planning and putting thought into your choice of goals, a number of relapses, the right type of motivation, and the self-confidence that you can do it. Incorporating new positive habits is no easy task, however, we can elevate our chances of successfully implementing new positive behaviours by examining the research. Below are some tips right from the literature on designing habits that stick:

- **Make habits fun:** For example, trampolining to get in exercise as opposed to joining a gym. The more fun, the better! This increases our levels of 'quality' motivation as we are doing a new behaviour we inherently enjoy.
- **Starting small so you can realistically achieve your habit:** When we feel good at achieving our goal, however small, we are much more likely to continue!
- **Break down larger goals into manageable small ones:** This ensures we don't feel overwhelmed.
- **Temptation bundling:** Linking pleasurable temptations with a habit that provides delayed rewards, such as only listening to your favourite podcast whilst cycling. This term was first coined by Katy Milkman (Milkman et al. 2014) after studying temptation bundling with behaviour change. This technique makes activities that have delayed rewards more enticing and much more readily executed. In a recent large study (n = 6792), participants took part in a four-week exercise programme (Kirgios et al. 2020). They received either an audiobook with advice to temptation bundle, only an audiobook, or neither. The results showed that giving participants audiobooks and encouraging temptation bundling increased their chances of a weekly workout by 10–14% and average weekly workouts by 10–12% 17 weeks postintervention.
- **Habit stacking:** Piggybacking off existing habits, such as adding a two-minute mindfulness breathing routine to a regular running habit.
- **Accountability buddy:** Adopting a friend or loved one to help you stay on track can be hugely effective.

- **Growth mindset approach:** New habits take time and persistence. Having a growth mindset, one that believes you can learn and grow, no matter what age, is hugely beneficial in helping you persist.
- **Fresh starts:** Hanging a habit change to different life chapters – that is, natural break points in life, such as a new move, starting a new job, the start of the week, or a new year.
- **Celebrate progress:** Increasing one's levels of positive emotions makes us feel good and more likely to continue with our habit. Acknowledging progress also helps you to lean towards a growth mindset.

Summary

- The 'quality' of motivation is more important than the type of motivation.
- Self-confidence is important in creating habits that stick.
- We can increase self-confidence by finding a mentor, using self-compassion and positive affirmations, and managing negative emotions (by mindfulness, self-compassion, and CBT).
- There are six stages to creating a new behaviour.
- Expect relapse when making a new behaviour, reward progress, and adopt growth mindset.
- The type of goals we set are important; we can use emotion to increase our motivation, ensure goals are clear and challenging, receive feedback, and break goals down into smaller, subgoals.
- Tips to build habits that stick: adopt a growth mindset, make it fun, keep small, celebrate, stack onto existing habits, bundle temptation, use fresh starts, and use an accountability buddy.

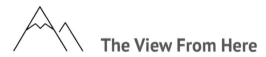 **The View From Here**

Think about the resolutions you formed this year: to eat better, to exercise more, to start mindfulness, and to practise gratitude. We know these things will benefit us enormously, but why is it that we abandon these habits within a few short weeks? Well, change is hard.

In this chapter, we explored how we can draw on the science of behavioural change to design a different path, by increasing our 'quality' motivation by supporting our sense of choice and freewill, becoming competent and mastering new tasks, and learning to support from mentors and family and friends. We can look to increase our self-confidence in achieving habits that stick by observing role models, using positive inner language, reflecting on past positive experiences, and managing negative thoughts that hijack our brain. We can also choose goals in a different way – one that stems from drawing on our emotions and values. Using these mind tools, we can *engineer* a life where we increasingly do what is good for us.

References

Bandura, A. (1977). Self-efficacy: toward a unifying theory of behavioral change. *Psychological Review* 84 (2): 191.

Deci, E.L. and Ryan, R.M. (1985). *Intrinsic Motivation and Self-Determination in Human Behavior*. New York: Plenum.

Deci, E.L. and Ryan, R.M. (2000). The 'what' and 'why' of goal pursuits: human needs and the self-determination of behavior. *Psychological Inquiry* 11: 227–268.

Duckworth, A.L. (2006). Intelligence is not enough: non-IQ predictors of achievement. Doctoral dissertation. University of Pennsylvania.

Kirgios, E.L., Mandel, G.H., Park, Y. et al. (2020). Teaching temptation bundling to boost exercise: a field experiment. *Organizational Behavior and Human Decision Processes* 161 (Supplement): 20–35.

Locke, E.A. (1968). Toward a theory of task motivation and incentives. *Organizational Behavior and Human Performance* 3: 157–189.

Locke, E.A. and Latham, G.P. (1990). *A Theory of Goal Setting and Task Performance*. Englewood Cliffs, NJ: Prentice Hall.

Milkman, K.L., Minson, J.A., and Volpp, K.G.M. (2014). Holding the hunger games hostage at the gym: an evaluation of temptation bundling. *Management Science* 60 (2): 283–299.

Prochaska, J.O. and DiClemente, C.C. (1983). Stages and processes of self-change of smoking: toward an integrative model of change. *Journal of Consulting and Clinical Psychology* 51 (3): 390–395.

13

The Road Ahead

This last well-being workout brings together the chapters exploring each pillar and helps you integrate everything in a practical way. Consider how you can boost your PERLE levels by filling out the final worksheet, *Boost Your PERLE Levels*.

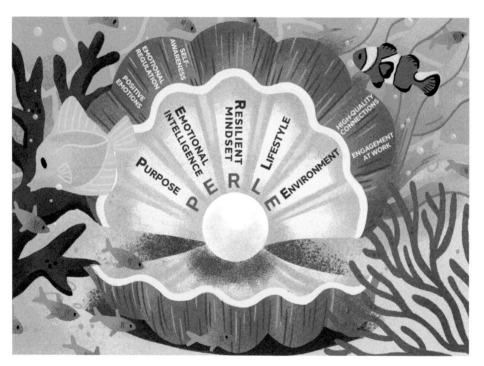

The PERLE Resilience Framework

Resilience and Well-being for Dental Professionals, First Edition. Mahrukh Khwaja.
© 2023 John Wiley & Sons Ltd. Published 2023 by John Wiley & Sons Ltd.
Companion website: www.wiley.com/go/khwaja-resilience-dentistry

P *Purpose*	Meaning at work, alignment with a greater purpose than ourselves. Understanding our core values as dental professionals, value-based goals, acts of kindness.
E *Emotional intelligence*	Understanding our emotions and the emotions of others, regulating our emotions, and harnessing the power of positive emotions.
R *Resilient mindset*	Thinking styles that are optimistic, compassionate, and growth.
L *Lifestyle*	Positive health including good nutrition, sleep, and movement.
E *Environment at work*	Positive and compassionate work cultures, high-quality connections, positive relationships, using strengths at work, getting in 'flow' states.

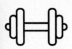

Boost Your PERLE Levels

1. Use the table below to think about each strand of the PERLE model. How do you fare according to each ingredient? Give each part of PERLE a score from 1–10 (10 being a lot).

2. Next, using the prompts below, fill out the blank table on the following page. Think of examples of how you can integrate more PERLE that helps you feel fulfilled, feel able to manage stressors, feel good, prioritise physical health, feel connected to others, and feel engaged at work.

3. Use this table as a reminder of your personalised resilience boosters and positive actions you can take to prioritise your well-being.

Purpose	**Emotional intelligence**	**Resilient mindset**	**Lifestyle**	**Environment**
Rating/10	*Rating/10*	*Rating/10*	*Rating/10*	*Rating/10*
• How can I bring my values to work and home? • How can I align my goals with my values? • What pursuits bring me meaning and make me feel worthwhile? For example, engaging in spiritual activities, fundraising, mentoring, teaching.	• Reflect on activities that could increase self-awareness, for example, a mindful check-in or journaling. • Consider activities that could help regulate stressors, such as mindfulness or self-compassion. • Consider what activities make you feel good.	• How can I reframe situations with optimism? • How can I lean into a compassionate mindset in response to stress and a harsh inner critic? • How can I move towards growth mindset when upskilling?	• How can I prioritise good nutrition this week? • Which activities do I enjoy that invite more movement? How can I do these more? • Which sleep hygiene tips can I apply to enjoy better and more sleep?	• When, where, and how I increase high-quality connections at work. • Who brings me joy and support? How can I amplify the positive in them? • How can I use my strengths at work and at home? • What activities help me get in the 'flow' and make me lose track of time?

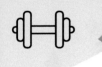

Boost Your PERLE Levels

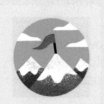

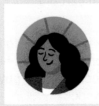

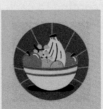

Recommendations for Change

To address the growing mental health crisis within dentistry, preventative action needs to be taken not only by the individual but by the dental team and the wider dental healthcare system. Table 13.1 summarises practical actions for positive well-being changes in dentistry.

Table 13.1 Practical action points for well-being changes in dentistry.

Change makers	Practical action points
Dental teams	• Identify mental well-being issues in the workplace early through adopting a **mental health lead**, who is trained in mental health first aid and suicide awareness, and design a work well-being action plan, as per the recommendations in the Dental Professional Alliance's *Mental Health Wellness in Dentistry Framework* (https://mhwd.org/framework/). In addition to the DPA's recommendation of stress management training for the team, I recommend **annual psychological resilience and well-being training** for all dental team members. Training should **not solely target addressing negative well-being markers (stress, anxiety, burnout) but should also foster positive well-being markers, such as resilience, increasing engagement at work, happiness, and quality of life**
	• Teams to support their staff through allocating protected space to complete well-being training courses.
	• Key performance indicators for dental teams to include well-being.
	• Integrating evidence-based well-being strategies into daily practice to foster kind, compassionate team cultures. Examples include:
	Mindful two minutes: Incorporate team mindfulness in a morning huddle or team debrief at the end of a clinical day.
	High-quality connections: Take moments in the day to prioritise positive relationships, through regular check-ins and mindful interactions with colleagues. Be compassionate and empathetic and celebrate positive aspects of each other's day by asking what went well for you today. To counteract loneliness and support professional development, include team-bonding days, mentorship, coaching, joining local peer support groups, and community interaction as part of a team well-being plan.
	Gratitude: Have regular appreciation conversations with team members, create a team gratitude board, or use gratitude in morning team huddles. The team can share positive comments from patients or treatment that has gone well.
	Strengths: Well-being training to include increasing engagement at work through strengths awareness and strengths spotting. Wherever possible, management to job craft to allow dental professionals to use their character strengths at work.

Table 13.1 (Continued)

Change makers	Practical action points
Dental governing bodies, for example, General Dental Council	• Spotlight clinician well-being through encouraging clinicians to complete courses and training as part of suggested CPD, in the same way medical emergencies, infection control, safeguarding children, and vulnerable adults and radiology are mandatory.
Dental trade unions	• Dental trade unions to continue to focus on improving working conditions for dental professionals, such as contract reforms and championing well-being CPD.
Dental education (undergraduate and postgraduate)	• Train university staff on student well-being and how to manage well-being concerns. • Integrate mandatory psychological resilience and well-being training into the dental curriculum for all dental students. • Design assessment tasks to increase student well-being as well as learning. • To increase uptake of mental health services and address stigma in dental students and postgraduates: targeted workshops on increasing awareness of how psychological and medical modalities can help boost your well-being. • Use of the **PERLE Resilience Model for Dental Professionals** to focus on the important pillars that can enhance resilience when designing psychological resilience workshops and programmes. • Develop psychological well-being programmes, workshops, and well-being conferences to be as available to dental professionals as clinical dentistry courses are.
Research and academia	• Create studies on the use of well-being interventions in dental professionals to help them thrive. • Interventions should **address increasing positive well-being markers, such as positive emotions, resilience, and engagement at work**, rather than a sole focus on reducing negative well-being markers. • Future research should also consider effects of varying culture and background on reported outcomes.
Government bodies, for example, Care Quality Commission	• National government bodies who inspect and regulate health services, such as the UK's Care Quality Commission, to make well-being a cornerstone of their assessment. This may include asking questions regarding whether staff feel supported by management and whether there is a designated well-being lead, and documenting what positive changes they have implemented based on this.

A Final Word

As busy dental professionals, working so closely with our patients and colleagues, we are at a greater risk of specific occupational hazards, such as burnout and compassion fatigue. The causes are multifactorial, and hence the solutions for poor mental well-being certainly need to be multipronged also. Fortunately, preventive education showcased in this book may bring the profession tremendous benefits. Drawing from the research into interventions for medical and healthcare professionals, we know that *intentional* well-being activities, whether that be mindful meditation, gratitude journaling, creating micro-moments of connection, forest bathing, cognitive reframing, or small acts of kindness, may buffer us against poor mental health outcomes, boost our positive emotions and resilience, increase our life satisfaction and meaning, and improve our relationships. To not just get to baseline but to move beyond it: to help you *thrive*. I hope these chapters have helped you to do just that – unpack the science of well-being and practically apply it to your work with patients and outside the clinic, so that you flourish in all areas of your life.

This book is designed to be a self-intervention, full of practical activities to boost your levels of positive feelings, positive thoughts, and positive actions. Experimentation of which well-being practices fit you the best will lead you to well-being practices that can be sustained long term. Your well-being experiments may include meditations, journaling, art therapy, and nature therapy. Furthermore, you may use the *Mental Wellness Check-in* as prompts to explore each facet of the PERLE model and apply it practically with your dental team or at home. Whatever experiments you try, keep self-compassion and growth mindset principles as your North Star: remind yourself that it's a journey, habits take time, and that how you talk to yourself in those moments makes all the difference to persevering.

Looking back on this well-being journey, which well-being practices resonate with you the most? For me, mindfulness and nature therapy bring me into my element. I get so much from this experience and feel so nourished. Far from just relaxation, mindfulness in nature increases my gratitude, compassion for others as well as myself, self-appreciation, and helps me set healthier boundaries with others, build a purpose-filled life, and provides greater clarity. Did integrating these well-being practices into my life solve all my problems? No, and that is not its aim. But I do know that my life is much more meaningful and richer because of making changes. I am a lot more alive, self-aware, and authentic because of it.

Going through this book, I hope you feel more optimistic about managing adversities and confident in your well-being strategies. I also hope you feel strengthened by the knowledge that resilience, along with all muscles of the mind, can be exercised and increased at any age. The first time I thought about this, and also learnt about neuroplasticity, I felt such relief. Knowing that we are not fixed to any capability was deeply exhilarating.

I hope the well-being activities in this book help you feel more zest in your life, energised, and confident in your ability to tap into your internal mental reservoirs when the going gets tough. As Jon Kabat-Zinn (2013) puts it, 'you can't stop the waves, but you can learn to surf them'. Happy surfing!

Reference

Kabat-Zinn, J. (2013). *Full Catastrophe Living*. Bantam Dell Publishing Group.

Index

Note: Page numbers in *italic* indicate figures.
Page numbers in **bold** indicate tables.

Resilience and Well-being for Dental Professionals, First Edition. Mahrukh Khwaja.
© 2023 John Wiley & Sons Ltd. Published 2023 by John Wiley & Sons Ltd.
Companion website: www.wiley.com/go/khwaja-resilience-dentistry

Printed and bound by CPI Group (UK) Ltd, Croydon, CR0 4YY

27/10/2024

14580162-0001